St. Louis Community College

Forest Park
Florissant Valley
Meramec

Instructional Resources
St. Louis, Missouri

Michael J. Holosko, PhD
Marvin D. Feit, PhD
Editors

Health and Poverty

Health and Poverty

HAWORTH Health and Social Policy
Marvin D. Feit, PhD
Senior Editor

New, Recent, and Forthcoming Titles:

*Maltreatment and the School-Age Child: Developmental Outcomes
and System Issues* by Phyllis T. Howing, John S. Wodarski,
P. David Kurtz, and James Martin Gaudin, Jr.

Health and Social Policy by Marvin D. Feit and Stanley F. Battle

*Adolescent Substance Abuse: An Empirical Based Group
Preventive Health Paradigm* by John S. Wodarski
and Marvin D. Feit

*Long-Term Care: Federal, State, and Private Options
for the Future* by Raymond O'Brien and Michael Flannery

Health and Poverty by Michael J. Holosko and Marvin D. Feit

Health and Poverty

Michael J. Holosko, PhD
Marvin D. Feit, PhD
Editors

The Haworth Press
New York • London

The Haworth Press, Inc., 10 Alice Street, Binghamton, NY 13904-1580

Cover design by Marylouise E. Doyle.

Library of Congress Cataloging-in-Publication Data

Health and poverty / Michael J. Holosko, Marvin D. Feit, editors.
     p. cm.
    Includes bibliographical references and index.
    ISBN 0-7890-0149-7 (alk. paper)
    1. Poor—Medical care—United States. 2. Poor—Medical care—Canada. 3. Poverty—Health aspects—United States. 4. Poverty—Health aspects—Canada. I. Feit, Marvin D. II. Holosko, Michael J.
RA418.5.P6H385 1997
362.1′086′942—dc21
                                                  97-9585
                                                  CIP

CONTENTS

ABOUT THE EDITORS

Michael J. Holosko, PhD, MSW, is Professor at the School of Social Work, University of Windsor. He has taught social work and nursing and has been a consultant in the health and human services field for the past 17 years in Canada, the United States, Europe, Asia, and Australia. His specialty areas are clinical and program evaluation, administrative skills, and stress management. He has published numerous monographs, chapters, and articles, and has conducted research studies primarily in the areas of health care, social policy, and evaluation. His texts include *The Evaluation of Employee Assistance Programs* (The Haworth Press, Inc., 1988), *Social Work Practice in Health Care Settings* (Canadian Scholars' Press [CSP], 1989), and *Social Work Practice with the Elderly* (CSP, 1991 and 1996). He is also on the editorial boards of the *Journal of Health and Social Policy,* the *Journal of Human Behavior in the Social Environment,* and the *Hong Kong Journal of Social Work.* He has served on numerous boards of directors for a variety of local, provincial, federal, and international human service agencies, including Health and Welfare Canada's Research Advisory Committee.

Marvin D. Feit, PhD, MSW, is Professor and Director of the School of Social Work at The University of Akron. He has taught social work graduate and undergraduate courses in administration and treatment, and has served as a consultant to a variety of health and human services organizations for the past 27 years. His areas of expertise are financial management, administration, group work, substance abuse, and health care. He has published many chapters, articles, monographs, and books over the years, including: The Management and Administration of Drug and Alcohol Programs; Evaluation of Employee Assistance Programs; Adolescent Substance Abuse; *Capturing the Power of Diversity;* Social Work Practice with the Elderly; and *Health and Social Policy.* He is also the founding editor of the *Journal of Health & Social Policy* published by The Haworth Press, Inc.

CONTRIBUTORS

Samuel L. Baker, PhD, is Assistant Professor, Department of Health Administration, School of Public Health, University of South Carolina.

Judith C. Barker, PhD, is affiliated with the Department of Epidemiology and Biostatistics, and with the Center for AIDS Prevention Studies at the University of California at San Francisco. She is also affiliated with the Department of Medical Anthropology Program, also at the University of California.

Robynn S. Battle, MPH, is affiliated with the Department of Epidemiology and Biostatistics, and with the Center for AIDS Prevention Studies at the University of California, San Francisco.

Cyril F. Chang, PhD, is Professor of Economics at Memphis State University, Memphis, Tennessee.

Valire Carr Copeland, PhD, MPH, is Assistant Professor, School of Social Work, the University of Michigan.

Gayle L. Cummings, MPH, is affiliated with the Department of Epidemiology and Biostatistics, and with the Center for AIDS Prevention Studies, at the University of California, San Francisco.

Susan E. Dawson, PhD, is Associate Professor, Department of Sociology, Social Work, and Anthropology, at Utah State University, Logan, Utah.

Loring Jones, DSW, is Assistant Professor of Social Work, School of Social Work, San Diego State University, San Diego, California.

Michele A. Kelley, MSW, ScD, is Assistant Professor of Community Health Sciences at the School of Public Health, the University of Illinois at Chicago.

Flora M. Krasnovsky, PhD, is affiliated with the Department of Epidemiology and Biostatistics, and the Center for AIDS Prevention Studies, at the University of California at San Francisco.

Jennie J. Kronenfeld, PhD, is Professor, School of Health Administration Policy, College of Business, Arizona State University.

Donald R. Leslie, PhD, is Assistant Professor, University of Windsor, School of Social Work, Windsor, Ontario, Canada.

Wangyue Liu, MS, is Research Specialist at the School of Public Health, the University of Illinois at Chicago.

Gary E. Madsen, PhD, is Associate Professor, Department of Sociology, Social Work, and Anthropology, at Utah State University, Logan, Utah.

Debra M. McPhee, MSc, is affiliated with the faculty of Social Work, University of Toronto, Ontario, Canada.

Naomi M. Morris, MD, MPH, is Professor and Director of Community Health Sciences at the School of Public Health, the University of Illinois at Chicago.

Patricia A. Nolan, MD, MPH, is currently Director of the Pima County Health Department, Tucson, Arizona. She is also a member of the adjunct faculty of the University of Arizona College of Medicine, in the Department of Family and Community Medicine.

Kant Patel, PhD, is Professor of Political Science, Southwest Missouri State University, Springfield, Missouri.

Janet D. Perloff, PhD, is Associate Professor at the School of Social Welfare and the School of Public Health, SUNY, Albany, New York.

Mitchell F. Rice, PhD, is Professor of Public Administration and Political Science at Louisiana State University, Baton Rouge. He has published extensively on public policy and minority health care issues. His most recent book is *Health Care Issues in Black America* (Greenwood Press, 1987) with Woodrow Jones Jr.

Madeleine R. Stoner, MSS, PhD, is affiliated with the University of Southern California School of Social Work, Los Angeles, California.

Howard P. Tuckman, PhD, is Distinguished Professor of Economics at Memphis State University, Memphis, Tennessee.

Preface

Since time immemorial, by virtue of their social status in any economic or political system, the poor represent the "have nots" of society. The extent to which any social or health care initiative can ameliorate the plight of the poor or lessen their stigmatization and victimization has been documented to be negligible. In North America, issues of poverty are ubiquitous and transcend any social and health care system. In truth, such issues effect the ways in which the provision and delivery of services are operationalized at all levels in the infrastructure from macro policy making to meso health care organizations to micro frontline providers.

This text is designed to sensitize readers to the health care realities of poverty in America today. It provides both the context for understanding the central issues underpinning any discussion of health and poverty and also the consequences or effects of such realities. We believe that such issues are of paramount importance and must not get lost in current discussions of reform or proposed changes in the health and medical care system. Indeed, while some of the chapters in this text were written in the context of national health care reform, the issues and concerns addressed by the authors remain central to the delivery of services and adequacy of care regardless of the outcome of any debate. The chapters in this text clearly support the contention that whether or not there is national health care reform, the poor will continue to be served differentially and unequally. That is, regional and economic disparity, unequal access to services, uneven quality of care, and discrimination will continue to prevail. In this regard, this text focuses attention on these concerns, and attempts to determine whether any services or programs can be provided to at least achieve more humane outcomes than currently exist.

A primary assumption of the *Journal of Health & Social Policy* (from which these chapters were collected and edited) is that health policy is intertwined with social policy. From a societal perspective then, how we care for the health of our nation is by its very nature indicative of how we care for the welfare of the nation. As a result, health policies are inextricably linked foremost to political agendas, economic priorities, and social and cultural values. Ironically, as we come to research and understand poverty in North American society, it is the latter point—namely, our prevailing social and cultural values—that present the greatest challenge toward developing competent, accessible, and affordable health care that may better meet or serve the needs of the poor.

Part I of this text, *The Context of Health Care Policies and Services*, provides the political and economic context for understanding health care policy issues and concerns related to the poor in the United States and Canada. McPhee, while reviewing the various health care reform proposals, concludes that the United States continues to focus on *who* receives medical care rather than *how* medical care is delivered and/or received. In the United States, she notes that receiving medical care is based on socioeconomic and/or employment status and contends that universal health care can result only when reform proposals are rejected which divide the populace into the "deserving" and "undeserving" categories.

Patel provides an historical perspective of the Medicaid program with emphasis on how the major changes in the 1980s impacted the states. He illustrates how decentralization of the Medicaid program gave state governments greater flexibility to tinker with new approaches in delivering health care to the poor. Nolan then provides a compelling argument for the delivery of primary prevention initiatives for the poor by highlighting structural conflicts existing between the health and welfare system in the state of Arizona. Jones explores the profound relationship between unemployment and health, since the former has been shown to be a stressful life event with severe health consequences. He notes that the health risks for the unemployed are likely to continue to be high or increase because we will enter future economic downturns with higher numbers of people out of work, and those who do lose their jobs will find less support from government and other arenas. The concluding chapter underscores the pervasive nature of North American poverty, as Leslie illustrates how the dichotomy between rich and poor pervades the national insurance program in Canada. Thus, a strong note of caution is raised for those who believe that a universal or national health system will better address the health care needs of the poor.

In Part II, titled *Impacts, Influences, Results, and Consequences*, Tuckman and Chang's lead chapter poses the poignant question, "Who bears the burden of uncompensated hospital care?" These authors suggest that the hospitals which provide services received by indigent patients may not bear the financial burden for such care. Subsequentally, they present a compelling argument identifying how indigent patients are unfairly and unequally treated in the existing health care system—just because they are poor. Rice's chapter reiterates this reality and describes the appropriately termed "patient dumping" phenomena, which usually occurs with indigent persons in emergency rooms all across America. He concludes that economic rather than medical reasons are the motivation for patient dumping, which in turn, exacerbates both the costs and provision of care for such persons. He then proposes that states should enact statutes "with teeth" to curtail this activity.

Copeland demonstrates that despite a consensus among policymakers, physicians, child health advocates, and the general public on the need to improve the overall health care delivery system, realistically few initiatives have taken place. She presents the Early and Periodic Screening Diagnosis and Treatment (EPSDT) program as an example of a national cost-effective strategy that can be used effectively to impact maternal and child health care services. She suggests that this program may help to alleviate the financial, systemic, and knowledge barriers which currently exist in providing health care for poor children.

Stoner provides national prevalence data on HIV/AIDS among homeless people, but focuses on the inequities of care as well as the barriers to health care for this population. She provides a prescription for a series of low-cost, pragmatic intervention strategies, and truly doubts whether federal, state, or local constituents will ever take such initiatives seriously given their track records to date.

Battle, Cummings, Barker, and Krasnovsky focus on an understudied population subjected to three abject determinants—gender, race, and poverty. Besides presenting data on HIV/AIDS African-

American low-income women who were part of the Parent Health Project, they focus on barriers to conducting research with such "hard to reach" populations, obstacles to care and provision of services, and the effectiveness of this particular program. They clearly reveal the very real difficulties and challenges of implementing such programs at the "grassroots level" in which they may have the greatest potential impact.

Kelley, Perloff, Morris, and Liu illustrate how many African-American infants and children lack access to primary care physicians or services in the Chicago region. Specifically, they lack regular and competent sources of care and prevention—despite the espoused national priorities for reducing infant mortality and proposing health development over the first year of life. In short, the national agenda has failed dismally for the African-American community. Baker and Kronenfeld provide an excellent example of referring high risk women and newborns to designated clinics in South Carolina for prenatal and newborn care. They present empirical evidence showing that effective screening and channeling of these patients leads to positive health outcomes. Dawson and Madsen provide a vivid account of some of the physical and emotional health effects of uranium milling on American Indian millworkers—a unique group that had never been studied before. Their exploratory study illustrates the impact of difficult and poor working conditions on the physical and emotional health of a low-income minority population, buried deep in the quagmires of the U.S. health care system.

PART I:
THE CONTEXT OF HEALTH CARE
POLICIES AND SERVICES

As the issue of health care reform currently hovers on the political horizon in North America, a major aspect of any initiative which strives for universal coverage is the inclusion of poor people. Part I provides the context for understanding the complex relationship between health care policies and services, and poverty. The chapters examine the inherent structural problems in attaining universal coverage; the Medicaid program; and the consequent health problems that result when people are unemployed and/or are poor. However, an examination of one universal health care program reveals that economic differences remain an intractable problem. Thus, there is no easy solution to meeting the health care needs of poor people, and poverty is arguably the single most important determinant of health status.

Chapter 1

Health Care in the United States: The Battle of Reform

Debra M. McPhee

INTRODUCTION

The word crisis has frequently been used to describe the current state of the American health care system. The majority of writers on the subject agree on the paramount crisis issues: escalating health care costs; inadequate coverage; relatively high levels of public dissatisfaction; and expensive, complex administrative requirements. There is, however, much less agreement on what should be done in the way of reform.

Proposals for health care reform generally fall into three categories: (1) private marketplace insurance; (2) employer-based health insurance; (3) centralized or single-payer health care models. This chapter will examine the current nature of the U.S. health care debate. Included is a critical review of the prominent health care reform proposals as they relate to issues of coverage, access to care, and the management of costs. The examination considers the influence of public opinion on the development of public health policy, and provides a critical analysis of some of the salient political issues likely to affect the future direction of the national health care debate in the United States.

THE STRUCTURE OF THE U.S. HEALTH CARE SYSTEM

Mapping the structure of the U.S. health care system is a challenging task. In theory, health care coverage is available to virtually

This chapter was originally published in *Journal of Health and Social Policy*, Vol. 7(1) 1995.

all Americans through one of four routes: (1) Medicare for the elderly and disabled; (2) Medicaid for low-income/public assisted individuals and persons with certain disabilities; (3) employer-subsidized coverage in the workplace; or (4) self-purchased coverage available through private insurance companies (e.g., Blue Cross/Blue Shield). A few additional sources of health care coverage do exist for special category individuals which include medical services provided to members of the Armed Services, and Veterans Administration (VA) medical programs. Each form of provision differs regarding eligibility requirements and the specific care aspects that are covered. The financing and administration of the various forms of health care are handled by way of a complicated patchwork of federal, state, and local legislation. Thus, the health care delivery "system" as it presently operates is in fact a complex, multilayered industry—an industry which has been plagued by a decade of rising costs and increasingly restrictive governmental policies resulting in a limiting of resources and service availability.

NATURE OF THE U.S. HEALTH CARE CRISIS

Coverage

It is estimated that between 31 to 37 million Americans are currently lacking some form of private or public medical insurance coverage.[1] While in excess of 33 million persons are presently enrolled in the Medicare program, coverage often becomes problematic when the physician bills the patient for more than the Medicare approved charge, leaving the patient liable for the difference.[2] In addition, the minimum deductibles and co-insurance amounts that the Medicare beneficiary must pay out-of-pocket can be substantial. With specific reference to public health assistance the Medicaid program has increasingly failed to provide adequate coverage to the persons it was designed to protect. The number of persons covered by this program has risen over the past decade from 30 to 37 million at the same time that the percentage of the poor *not* covered by Medicaid has risen from about 35% to about 60%.[3]

Americans who do not qualify for health care coverage through either the Medicare or Medicaid programs, and are not covered by way of employer-assisted plans, are left with the option of securing adequate coverage for themselves and their families through one of the many private health insurance companies. Presently, consumers must choose from among the 1,500 private insurance companies operating throughout the United States. Each company is free to specify its own eligibility requirements, extent of coverage, and reimbursement rates. Insurance premiums are, of course, the responsibility of the individual, and vary widely from company to company.

As with any other consumer good, purchasing health insurance in a private marketplace system means one generally gets what one pays for. Insurance packages that provide anything above a minimum level of coverage are often costly and beyond the financial resources of most Americans. With health care costs on the rise, many private insurance companies have begun to institute strict eligibility requirements, restricting types and amounts of coverage offered, and have significantly increased their premiums. Consequently, even those persons who do manage to retain coverage may find themselves without enough coverage at a time of illness or injury. It is estimated that well over 50 million persons in the United States are inadequately covered by their present health insurance, meaning that a major illness will translate into almost certain financial ruin.[4]

As an alternate choice, Health Maintenance Organizations (HMOs) have been presented as the solution to the health care crisis in general and to the problems of the Medicare/Medicaid programs in particular. It has been argued that incorporating HMOs into Medicaid would improve the states' abilities to budget expenditures, simplify management, eliminate abusive practices directly linked to fee-for-service care, and contain costs.[5] It has further been argued that increasing the use of HMOs will increase general access to mainstream medicine.[6] But while alternative structures such as HMOs continue to enjoy support, they have also been severely criticized for illustrating poor program designs, unethical marketing practices, inadequate or underservicing, and excessive administrative costs.[7]

In the past, coverage for American workers, and often their dependents, was a cornerstone of health insurance. In recent years, however, employer-subsidized health insurance plans have suffered greatly. Since the early 1980s it is estimated that the percentage of corporate profits consumed by health care has risen from 29% to

49%.[8] In response to continually rising costs many employers have reduced the amount of health care coverage they offer or have canceled employee insurance benefits altogether. Even when employers do not restrict health care coverage, an increasing number of insurance companies are excluding individuals based on prior health conditions, and some exclude entire industries whose employees are considered "high risk." Consequently, employment alone does not necessarily guarantee greater access to health care coverage and many of the "working poor" across the United States do not receive adequate medical treatment. Ironically, the nonworking poor may, in some cases, receive better medical care than their employed counterparts. For example, an unemployed poor person may be eligible for Medicaid benefits or indigent care, whereas an employed poor person may be denied benefits or indigent care precisely because he or she is employed. In brief, the working poor fall between the cracks—they have too little income to purchase adequate health insurance and too much income to qualify for medical assistance. Thus, with respect to health care coverage there exists great disparity in the U.S. system. At one extreme, active duty military personnel receive complete medical coverage; at the other end, well over 14% of the population receive little or no medical coverage.

Access to Care

On a state-by-state comparison the proportion of uninsured varies depending on several factors, including the level of Medicaid coverage in the state, the demographics of the population, insurance practices, overall income, the nature of employment, and the individual state health policy. Of those clients who are covered by Medicaid, access to care is not necessarily guaranteed. While care is theoretically available, health care facilities are frequently so overloaded that access is unrealistic. Again, while Medicaid patients theoretically have the option of choosing their own physicians, in reality the choice is not the recipients'. More and more physicians have refused to accept Medicaid clients. Physicians' resistance to treating such patients has been ascribed to many causes, including low and delayed Medicaid payments, fears of malpractice litigation, paperwork, cultural or language problems, noncompliance, and other factors, including racial discrimination.[9] Undoubtedly, the prospect of low or nonexistent payment is a disincentive to most providers who, under the guidelines set down by the American Medical Association, have the right to refuse treatment if the patient cannot demonstrate an ability to pay up-front.[10] Thus, a complete health care screening in the United States includes a specific evaluation of a person's ability to pay *before* he or she can receive care. Many cannot measure up and as a result it is estimated that every year more than 1 million American citizens are turned away by health care practitioners and institutions because they lack financial means or medical coverage.[11]

Health Care Spending and the Issue of Cost

The issue of cost and the need for cost containment with respect to health care spending is most often the primary focus of the health care debate. Unquestionably the cost of health care in all the industrialized countries is high and rising fast. Since the early 1970s the percentage of the U.S. GNP consumed by health care has continued to rise to well over 12%.[12] Interestingly, the percentage of the GNP consumed by health care costs for both the United States and its closest neighbor, Canada, was virtually identical (around 9%) until 1971, when Canada adopted a centralized national health insurance plan.[13] Since that time Canadian percentages have stayed around 9% while the U.S. figures have continued to climb. In just one decade U.S. annual health care spending has increased from $248 billion to $650 billion.[14] This means the United States currently spends over $3,000 per person, per year, in a system which still leaves one in four persons uninsured or without adequate health insurance coverage.[15]

Public health programs, and specifically the Medicaid program, have long been primary targets of governmental cost containment initiatives in the health care field. In the early 1980s under the Reagan administration, both the federal and state governments sought to control or reduce Medicaid expenditures in the face of tax cuts, growing costs, and reduced federal funds for the program. This led to freezes and reductions in both eligibility and provider payments. The result was a basically stable number of beneficiaries despite an increase in the poverty population.[16] Thus the health care cutbacks and cost containment measures of both the Reagan and Bush administrations resulted in decreased access and eligibility for persons in need, without significantly reducing the overall cost of health care delivery.

Social Implications

Although inadequate health care may bring personal tragedy to impoverished individuals, the long-term consequences may be even more costly to the society as a whole. The National Center for Health Statistics reports that in 1988, 17% of American children under the age of 18 years had neither private insurance nor Medicaid coverage.[17] Given the numerous studies validating the importance of preventative medical treatment and early intervention, particularly with respect to prenatal care, these rates are, at the very least, alarming.

Studies have consistently shown that babies born to mothers with no prenatal care are five times more likely to die and three times more likely to end up in neonatal intensive care units.[18] The United States, the same country that ranks number one in the world for health care spending, presently ranks twentieth in the world in infant mortality.[19] The maintenance of a system that fails to focus on prevention as a medical priority has a great deal to do with this situation. Statistics indicate that while 95% of Canadian women will receive prompt prenatal care, this is true for only about 75% of pregnant women in the United States.[20] Currently, a baby born in Detroit, Michigan is 38% more likely to die in the first year of life than a baby born just across the border in Windsor, Ontario.[21] Clearly preventative medical services do not come cheaply. However, while Canada may be ranked number two in the world in health care spending, it also boasts the second highest life expectancy rate at birth for both sexes and has the second lowest infant mortality rate, next to Japan.[22]

Although health care coverage in itself is not the sole determinant of health status, Medicaid data has repeatedly demonstrated that coverage is a key factor in overall health and well-being.[23] And although availability of care does not in and of itself guarantee improved health, medical indigence has been strongly associated with lack of care and poor health status. What is clear, is that presently the uninsured represent significant costs both economically and socially. While most of the uninsured will receive acute care services in necessary situations, the point of entry into the system is generally at the worst stage—through the hospital emergency room. Here it is often a case of too little too late with the results generally being high costs and poor outcomes. Furthermore, it is increasingly the case that preventable conditions are being treated as emergency cases in the least cost-effective manner, with hospitals having to provide primary care in their emergency settings.

Clearly the impact of the U.S. health care crisis can be felt in every sector, both public and private. The nature of the health care crisis for the individual American is essentially identical to that of the nation as a whole—restricted accessibility and the high and uncertain costs of obtaining medical care. In recent years pressure on the government to reform the health care system has escalated, coming mainly from the inadequately covered, employers, big business, and employee groups. Further, there is a growing consensus that the incremental reform efforts of the past are no longer sufficient for bringing about the level of fundamental change required.

PROPOSALS AND PROMISES OF REFORM

For the better part of a decade, "reform" of the U.S health care industry has meant the introduction of governmental cost containment initiatives and increased regulatory policies which have meant an inevitable partial abandonment of traditional American free market policies. Proposals supporting employer-mandated insurance plans are on the rise, and in recent years considerable attention has been devoted to arguments that the time has come for the United States to adopt a more efficient and equitable national single-payer health care plan. With the emphasis on systematic reform, the sense of urgency and need to find solutions has been extended from the state to the national level, and there exists no shortage of proposals or opinions. Proposals for health care delivery and reform generally fall into three categories: (1) private marketplace or third-party payment plans; (2) employer-based health care plans; and (3) single-payer or centrally administered plans. Most would agree that the basic principles of equity and efficiency should be central objectives of any new health care scheme to be considered. However, as one sifts through myriad reform proposals it is clear that there is considerable variability when it comes to definitions and how the ideals of *equity* and *efficiency* are to be achieved.

The Private Marketplace and the Third-Party Payer

Defenders of the current free market system are prepared to argue that with respect to the purchase of goods and services it is the consumers who know best what they want and what they need. It is argued that the very structure of the competitive marketplace will force insurance and health service providers to keep costs down and quality high. Educated consumers are free to make informed decisions regarding health care plans and in return the insurance companies, forced to stay competitive, will empower consumers by providing the best service at the lowest prices possible.

Yet as one listens closely to the arguments of those Americans who support the current practices, there seems to be little attention paid to the portion of the population who, even if they are capable of selecting from among the hundreds of companies and wading through the complex insurance information, still find themselves without the financial resources necessary to purchase adequate health plans. With regards to disadvantaged groups or individuals it has been recommended that the government offer a certain amount of tax credits as a way of extending health care coverage. The basic assumption seems to be that any social problems encountered or created will be solved by the efficacy of the market. Rarely are the problems of the underinsured, or the fact that since 1971 the cost of individual health care has risen 168% while the rise in "real" wage has risen only 1%, adequately addressed.[24] Moreover, there are few solutions, if any, offered for how best to deal with the costly and complicated administrative problems which have become a trademark of third-party payment systems. By way of illustration, although Americans spend more on health care than their Canadian neighbors, Canadians receive more service for every health care dollar they spend.[25] It is estimated that approximately *half* the cost differential between the two nations can be attributed to the tremendous overhead and administrative costs of the American system.[26] Yet, organizations such as the Health Insurance Association of America continue to support the current administrative arrangements claiming that they serve a necessary policing function of health care providers.[27]

By definition, those who endorse the privatization of health care support a multilayered system where access to service is dependent heavily on one's financial resources. While it is argued that the free market approach is the answer to the problems of rising costs, the strength of this position has been weakened considerably by the fact that the third-party payment system presently in operation in the United States has failed to demonstrate this ability.

Employment-Based Health Care Plans

Historically, American labor and union leaders have maintained employee health benefits on the agenda of contract negotiations. But as Frishof[28] points out, the cost crisis of the 1980s "took away the first-dollar coverage previously enjoyed by many members of the stronger unions." Thus, as the costs continued to rise, the late 1980s saw unions being pressured into larger and larger givebacks. Today, employer-mandated health insurance proposals are plentiful, having received serious attention through the work of several influential interest groups. Such plans promote that universal coverage can be obtained by promoting existing insurance plans and requiring employers to insure all their workers. Expansion of public programs is the recommendation most frequently offered for extending health care benefits to the unemployed. However, employer-mandated plans have been challenged on many counts and some have asserted that such plans are no more than a polite guise for profoundly regressive health care financing.[29]

First, under such plans coverage may vary widely depending on the resources of the employer and the insurance plan selected. Clearly, large corporations have the advantage over small business employers in their ability to offer more comprehensive health benefits to their employees. Being in a position to offer more extensive plans means larger organizations are often able to attract and retain personnel better than their smaller competitors. Second, it is argued that employers forced to provide costly health benefits are likely to shift the costs back to their employees in the form of income restrictions and wage reductions. With health care coverage being so dependent on one's place of employment, an individual's mobility and freedom to move between companies or careers become extremely limited.

Third, employer-mandated health care programs often serve to foster discriminatory practices by employers. Employees are likely to be subjected to rigorous medical evaluations as a prerequisite to employment, with many individuals being disqualified based on factors such as their present states of health or interpretations of their medical histories. Women in particular may be vulnerable, with many employers concerned that women employees will "drain" health benefit resources by becoming pregnant and having children during the courses of their employment. Most important, placing the responsibility for solving the problems of the health care system on the shoulders of small business once again fails to address the fundamental problems at the core of the system which are driving the costs up in the first place. Employer-based health care plans are simply another means of making a person's right to basic health and basic health care dependent on a person's level of income and worth in the workplace.[30] Attempting to achieve universal coverage in this way is a contradiction, since truly universal programs are founded on the premise that all citizens of a society share the right to a basic standard of living and well-being regardless of position, and that a responsible society ensures equal access to key resources and services which help make this basic standard attainable.

The Nation As Single Payer

At present the United States and the Republic of South Africa are the only two countries in the industrialized world which do not have some form of national health insurance. In recent years U.S. governments have received increasing pressure from all segments of the society demanding fundamental reorganization of the current delivery system. Indeed, many reasonably argue that simply pouring more funds into the current system does not address the interdependent problems of rising costs and declining access.[31] Further, it is argued that incremental adjustments to the existing health care system (i.e., expansion of employer-based insurance and increased public funds to expand Medicaid) is an unrealistic long-term solution.[32]

Those who are in favor of the United States adopting national health insurance frequently present the Canadian model as a positive example of a centrally administered single-payer program. In brief, the structure and design of the Canadian national plan guarantees the principles of universality, comprehensive coverage, ease of access, public administration, portability, and a medical care program that covers 99% of the population.[33] The financing of the plan is provided by way of a governmental cost-sharing arrangement in which federal contributions and provincial taxes are provided in roughly equal proportion. Although each province is free to design its own system, the provincial programs must be compatible with federal guidelines to be eligible for the federal-provincial cost sharing. It is an important distinction that the health care system in Canada is not a monitored health service but rather an insurance program administered nationally and uniformly. Half of all hospitals in Canada are privately owned, and physicians are both salaried and reimbursed. Doctors receive a fee-for-service payment while government sets the fixed annual budgets for hospitals. Canadians are free to choose their doctors and the hospitals they use. Each person is issued a health insurance identification card by the province in which he or she lives. Most important, access to care is equally distributed and guaranteed regardless of individual income.

Certainly there is ample evidence that consolidation of purchasing power under a public agency is the most efficient way to free physicians from myriad administrative intrusions that currently plague the practice of medicine in the United States.[34] Presently administrative costs are five times greater in the United States than in Canada.[35] Nevertheless, proposals which suggest that the United States abandon its free market approach in favor of a Canadian-style universal government administered health care program have met with considerable opposition. There is a general consensus in the United States that the more government is involved, the more inefficient the plan and the more individual freedom will be restricted. However, this has not proven to be the case in the administration of the Canadian plan. American critics of universal insurance plans routinely argue that health care models such as Canada's involve resource rationing and the limiting of access to higher technologies. What is often not discussed is the fact that regardless of the specific system structure, health care services in *all* countries are rationed in some way and this includes the United States. The issue is not *if* rationing is necessary but rather *what kind* of rationing is preferable. The Canadian plan has often been criticized for its rationing of resources by limiting the availability of equipment and personnel, and for maintaining waiting lists for elective procedures. Most critics, however, fail to demonstrate that rationing access by way of equipment or personnel restrictions, for *nonemergency* conditions, results in any negative implications for health. Americans have chosen to ration resources by granting access to health equipment and services to those who are able to pay and by limiting access to those who cannot pay. The consequences of this form of rationing are profound. By way of example, the United States, the same country that leads the field in state-of-the-art medical technologies, currently has the poorest record of child immunizations and the highest rates of child tuberculosis in the Western world.[36]

Preliminary proposals from the Clinton Administration have served to escalate the debate over centralized national health insurance even further. Each group of health care analysts have become increasingly skilled at the art of manipulating statistics and rhetoric in the interest of supporting their position. As a result it has become increasingly difficult for the average American citizen to ascertain a realistic picture of the advantages, the disadvantages, and/or the feasibility of the reform proposals offered.

Public Policy and Public Opinion

It has been suggested that if public policy were determined solely by American public opinion polls, the United States would have had a universal health insurance plan years ago.[37] Comparing the U.S. and Canadian systems, a 1990 *Los Angeles Times* survey[38] found that most Americans (roughly 66% of those surveyed) would prefer the structure of the Canadian model to their current health care arrangements. Similarly a 1990 survey of ten countries[39] including the Netherlands, Italy, West Germany, France, Sweden, Australia, and Japan found that Canadians were the most satisfied with their current health care system while Americans were the least satisfied. Most significantly, even when asked to consider that a national health plan would be financed by an increase in taxes, between 60 and 70% of Americans choose the national health plan over the current system.[40]

For anyone who has followed the nature of the U.S. health care debate over the past decade these findings are hardly surprising. Yet, focusing on opinion poll results may serve only to distract from the more critical issues. In evaluating any health care delivery model, it is not so much satisfaction which is most important but whether or not the population as a whole enjoys a high level of health and well-being as a result of that model. Presently, this is not the case for a significant proportion of the American population. Numerous AMA-sponsored surveys[41] have reported that the American people, as well as American physicians, consider cost as the first concern facing the health care system today. Issues of accessibility are considered the second largest concern. Still, the country's inability to agree on any single reform approach simply reflects the indecisiveness created by the competing interests of national health organizations' leaders, service providers, and Congressional representatives.

THE POLITICS OF HEALTH CARE REFORM

The root of American resistance to fundamental reform may be found in the very social and political ideological fabric of society itself. The United States is a political democracy with a capitalist economy. Democracy implies equality at least with respect to the political process, however, at the same time capitalist economies promote inequality and, in fact, rely on it.[42] Thus, there is a blatant contradiction in a country that professes egalitarian political and social opportunity and yet maintains and generates gaping disparities in economic well-being. As has already been noted, nowhere are these disparities more glaring than within the health care sector.

Generally social welfare has been viewed by western industrialized countries as a necessary device for maintaining the social structure, strength, and well-being of the society as a whole. The United States, with its trillion-dollar economy, currently is among the richest countries in the world. No doubt other countries are mystified by the United States' position that it cannot afford increases in spending for social service improvements and in particular for improvements in health care. The paradox is striking, with the populace demanding increased and improved services on the one hand and tax cuts and increased private consumption on the other.

The United States has increasingly looked to private capital markets for sources of financing health care capital. Yet, if the health care system in the United States truly did operate as other consumer markets, then presumably the consumers (patient and potential patients) would play key roles as decision makers and the health care system would exist to serve both their wants and needs. Within the present health care system, consumers' needs and wants are, in large measure, defined for them. This is not to say that governments do not attempt to manage and direct the manner in which the system evolves. However, without a national approach, consistency among policies is lost as they are carried out among multiple agencies with differing organization, goals, and agendas. Therefore, government health care policy typically encompasses contradictions that reflect the many prominent interest groups that come to influence it. Likewise, planning within the current system is most often done at the individual hospital or hospital system level. Thus, a primary objective has naturally become the survival needs of for-profit organizations and securing the position of these institutions in the marketplace. Further, when a society chooses to treat health care as a consumer good rather than a community service, legitimate questions are raised regarding those who control the profits. Central questions focus on who should finance, own, and control the equipment and structures used in modern health care. In the United States American physicians rank prominently among health care industry investors.[43] By contrast Canada and most European nations have clearly decided that the capital used in health care should be financed and owned primarily by the public sector. Thus, health care capital is rarely owned by private investors and certainly not by physicians.

An examination of the interplay of social, political, and economic factors would suggest that it is not realistic to anticipate that the newly elected Clinton administration will be empowered to introduce any breakthrough health care reforms during its time in office. The ideological barriers to governmental involvement in the medical care market, public resistance to higher taxes and public spending, as well as competing priorities for the federal budget continue to present major road blocks. Battistella and Wheeler[44] predict that "while there will be an expansion of services in accord with the principle that access to them is a right, the economic and political realities point to incremental progress based on principles of plural-ism and selectivity rather than principles of universalism and ega-litarianism."

Given the political process prevailing in the United States, it is not surprising that there has been a trial-and-error approach to refor-mation of the health care system through marginal rather than radi-cal changes. It is logical to assume that the financial agendas of the major interest groups will continue to have a strong influence with respect to U.S. public policy formation. Within the domain of health policy, these interest groups have historically been the Medical Associations, multinational pharmaceutical companies, health care providers, and health insurers. While none of these groups is pow-erful enough by itself to directly dictate public health policy, com-bined they have demonstrated an ability to effectively veto any proposed legislation that they oppose. Reinhardt summarizes the American political climate most aptly when he notes, "In a society that views success and poverty as primarily the products of free choice rather than of mere fortune, the well-to-do are not easily moved to make sacrifices."[45]

CONCLUSION

There is little doubt that an era of inevitability is upon the United States with respect to health care reform. Over the past decade pressure has been exerted from many directions for an overhaul of the present system. While support for fundamental reform appears to be growing among the public and the policy makers alike, there remains a lack of consensus as to what shape the new system should take. The governmental cost containment measures of the 1980s have more often than not been unsuccessful in their prime objec-tive, and have served only to restrict further services to those most in need. In recent years there has been an increase in the number of advocates in favor of the United States adopting a plan of national health insurance, based on a centralized model. Yet there remains a significant number of powerful groups and individuals who oppose any scheme which would call for greater government involvement or restrictions which could potentially interfere with this enormous-ly profitable industry. As the Clinton administration attempts to aggressively tackle the problem, those most invested in maintaining the existing system will be busy renewing the strength of their opposition.

It has been demonstrated that there has yet to be developed a system without shortcomings or gaps in the "safety net." All countries utilizing some form of centralized universal health insurance also incorporate some means of rationing their resources. As costs continue to rise, countries supporting universal plans will need to be more efficient in *how* their medical care is delivered and received. The United States on the other hand, continues to focus on measures that propose being more selective about *who* receives medical care based on socioeconomic and/or employment status. The widespread negative consequences of this kind of selectivity have been clearly demonstrated with respect to the health status both of individual Americans and the nation as a whole. As social and economic conditions force Americans to rethink their current health delivery practices, government's success in securing universal health care for all citizens hinges on the extent to which it is willing to reject proposals which divide its populace into the "deserving" and the "undeserving."

NOTES

1. See Marmor, T. (1993). Commentary on Canadian Health Insurance: Lessons for the United States. *International Journal of Health Services*, 23(1), 45-62.; Reinhardt, U. (1992). Commentary: Politics and the Health Care System. *The New England Journal of Medicine*, 327(11), 809-811.; Woolhandler, S. et al. (1993). High Noon for U.S. Health Care Reform. *International Journal of Health Services*, 23(2), 193-211.

2. Renas, S., and Kinard, J. (1990). Importing the Canadian Plan. *Health Progress*, March, p. 23.

3. Inglehart, J. (1992). Health Policy Report. *The New England Journal of Medicine*, 327(20), 1467-1472.

4. Friedman, E. (1991). The Uninsured: From Dilemma to Crisis. *JAMA*, 19(May), p. 2492.

5. Spitz, B. (1979). When a Solution is Not a Solution: Medicaid and Health Maintenance Organizations. *Journal of Health Politics, Policy, and Law*, 3(4), 497-518.

6. Spitz, p. 498.

7. Spitz, p. 514.

8. Weisberg, R., and Mayers, L. (1990). Borderline Medicine. *PBS: Public Policy Productions*.

9. Fossett, J. W. et al. (1991). Medicaid Patients Access to Office Based Obstetricians, in Friedman, E. (1991). The Uninsured: From Dilemma to Crisis. *JAMA*, 19(May), p. 2492.

10. Relman, A., and Reinhardt, U. (1986). Debating For-Profit Health Care and the Ethics of Physicians. *Health Affairs* (Summer), p. 6.

11. Weisberg and Mayers.

12. Woolhandler, S. et al. (1993). High Noon for U.S. Health Care Reform. *International Journal of Health Services*, 23(2), 193-211.

13. Woolhandler et al.

14. Weisberg and Mayers.

15. Clinton, W. (1992). The Clinton Health Care Plan. *The New England Journal of Medicine*, 327(11), 804-807.

16. Friedman, p. 2492.

17. National Center for Health Services Research and Health Care Technology Assessment (1991). in Friedman, E. (1991). The Uninsured: From Dilemma to Crisis. JAMA, 19(May), p. 2491.

18. Weisberg and Mayers.

19. Weisberg and Mayers.

20. Weisberg and Mayers.

21. Weisberg and Mayers.

22. Mhatre, S., and Deber, R. (1992). From Equal Access to Health Care to Equitable Access to Health: A Review of Canadian Provincial Health Commissions and Reports. *International Journal of Health Services*, 22(4), p. 648.

23. Friedman, p. 2493.

24. Health Care Forum (April 1992). *Public Broadcasting Service*.

25. Health Care Forum.

26. Evans, R. (1988). Split Vision: Interpreting Cross-Border Differences in Health Spending. *Health Affairs*, 7(4), 17-24.

27. Weisberg and Mayers.

28. Frishof, K. (1990). Universal Access versus Universal Insurance. *Health Progress* (April), p. 53.

29. Woolhandler, S., p. 195.

30. Ehrenreich, B. (1992). Health Care Forum. *Public Broadcasting Service*.

31. See Cassidy, J. (1990). Health Care System Reform May Be on the Horizon. *Health Progress* (March), 27-29; Reinhardt, U. (1989). Commentary: Health Insurance for the Nation's Poor. *Health Affairs* (Spring), 101-109; and Himmelstein, D., and Woolhandler, S. (1986). Cost Without Benefit: Administrative Waste in US Health Care. *New England Journal of Medicine,* no. 314, 441-445.

32. Grumbach, K. et al. (1991). Liberal Benefits, Conservative Spending. *JAMA*, 265(19), p. 2553.

33. Mhatre and Deber, p. 646.

34. Grumbach, p. 2549.

35. Weisberg and Mayers.

36. Health Care Forum.

37. Navarro, V. (1989). Why Some Countries Have National Health Insurance, Others Have National Health Services, and the United States Has Neither. *International Journal of Health Services*, 19(3), p. 384.

38. Blendon, R. et al. (1990). Satisfaction with Health Systems in Ten Nations. *Health Affairs* (Summer), p. 187.

39. Blendon, R. et al.

40. Blendon, R., and Donelan, K. (1991). Interpreting Public Opinion Surveys. *Health Affairs* (Summer), p. 167.

41. Harvey, L.K. (1991). AMA Survey of Public and Physicians' Opinions on Health Care Issues. *American Medical Association*.

42. Davidson, S. (1980). *Medicaid Decisions: A Systematic Analysis of the Cost Problem*. Ballinger Publishing Co., p. 12.

43. Relman and Reinhardt.

44. Battistella, R., and Wheeler, J. (1978). *HealthCare Policy in a Changing Environment*. McCutchan Pub. Corp., p. 389.

45. Reinhardt, U. (1987). Health Insurance for the Nation's Poor. *Health Affairs* (Spring), p. 104.

Chapter 2

Medicaid:
Perspectives from the States

Kant Patel

INTRODUCTION

Two major developments occurred in the Medicaid program during the 1980s. First, in the early 1980s the Reagan administration introduced major changes designed to decentralize the Medicaid program. State governments were given more autonomy and flexibility to attempt innovative approaches to providing health care for the poor and also contain rising Medicaid costs. Second, beginning in 1984–1985, Democrats in Congress succeeded in imposing various mandates on the states designed to expand the Medicaid program coverage.

MEDICAID DECENTRALIZATION 1981–1984

The most important spending and policy shift affecting health care for the poor was incorporated in the *Omnibus Budget Reconciliation Act (OBRA) of 1981*. This legislation contained three major changes affecting the Medicaid program. First, the federal contribution to Medicaid was directly reduced—3% in 1982, 4% in 1983, and 4.5% in 1984. Second, changes in the federal welfare eligibility

This chapter was originally published in *Journal of Health and Social Policy*, Vol. 7(3) 1996.

policy reduced welfare rolls and thereby the number of eligible Medicaid recipients. Third, the law also contained many fundamental policy changes in Medicaid itself with far-reaching implications.[1] For example, although Medicaid had historically followed Medicare's reasonable cost reimbursement principle, the act allowed states to pay health care providers (hospitals, nursing homes) on a basis other than reasonable cost. The 1981 OBRA also authorized formal retreat from the principle of free choice with regard to provider eligibility. The Act gave states wide discretion, on approval from the Secretary of the Department of Health and Human Services (HHS), to limit Medicaid recipients' freedom to choose their doctors or hospitals. Other provisions made it easier to use new kinds of health care providers, particularly HMOs. The law also granted states wide discretion in deciding whom to cover under Medicaid. It also authorized a provision allowing payment, through a waiver from the Secretary of HHS, for a wide range of home and community services that states could cover as an alternative to nursing home care. The Act also allowed the states to buy laboratory services and medical devices via competitive bidding.

The *Tax Equity and Fiscal Responsibility Act of 1982* created new financing initiatives that allowed shifting costs to beneficiaries and third parties by granting the states discretion to require Medicaid beneficiaries to pay nominal fees for medical services.

The *Deficit Reduction Act of 1984* required Medicaid beneficiaries to assign to the states any rights they had to other health benefit programs. This allowed the states to collect from such programs any available payments for medical care for the covered beneficiaries.

MEDICAID EXPANSION 1984–1990

By 1984, Reagan initiatives to prune the Aid for Families and Dependent Children (AFDC) rosters were beginning to be challenged, and Congress began to ease eligibility standards. Since 1984 there have been many incremental expansions of the Medicaid program aimed primarily at covering more low-income pregnant women, infants, and children. Thus, for example, under the *Budget Reduction Act of 1984,* Congress required states to broaden their Medicaid coverage to include more low-income women during their first pregnancies, pregnant women in two-parent families in which the principal breadwinner was unemployed, and poor children up to the age of five in two-parent families.

The *Omnibus Budget Reconciliation Act of 1986* gave states the option to extend Medicaid coverage to pregnant women and infants up to age one and who were members of households with incomes of as much as 100% of the federal poverty level. The law also allowed coverage to be gradually implemented for children up to age eight in households with incomes less than the federal poverty level.

The *Omnibus Budget Reconciliation Act of 1987* allowed states to expand Medicaid eligibility to include pregnant women and infants up to age one and who were living in households with incomes of as much as 185% of the federal poverty level. States were also given the option of immediately covering all children younger than age five living in households with incomes less than the federal poverty level.

In 1988, Congress passed a law to help avoid impoverishing the spouses of patients who receive Medicaid financed nursing home care. The "spousal impoverishment" benefit—one of the few provisions to service the Medicare Catastrophic Coverage Act that was repealed in 1989—substantially raised the amount of income that a spouse could retain before handing the balance over to Medicaid to help defray the cost of a patient's nursing home care. The federal law allows states to let "at-home" spouses retain as much as $66,480 of the couple's combined assets and as much as $1,662 in monthly income.[2]

The *Omnibus Budget Reconciliation Act of 1989* required provision of all Medicaid-allowed treatment to correct problems identified during Early and Periodic Screening, Diagnosis, and Treatment (EPSDT), even if the treatment was otherwise not covered under the state Medicaid plan. The Act also required periodic screening under EPSDT if medical problems were suspected. The *Budget and Reconciliation Act of 1990* required Medicaid coverage of children under age 18 if the family income was below 100% of the federal poverty line.

President Reagan's New Federalism initiatives posed a new challenge to the health policies established over the last 50 years.[3] The Reagan administration was willing to grant states more discretion when such discretion promised cost reductions.[4] The New Federalism's emphasis on decentralization, combined with significant expansion of the program through federal mandates, raises a fundamental question: can the state governments contain dramatically rising costs and also provide access and quality care to the poor? How states respond to this challenge will shape the future course of Medicaid policy in particular and health care policy in general.

This chapter provides an analysis of how state governments responded to the Medicaid program's decentralization and expansion during the 1980s. The analysis is based on a survey of state Medicaid directors. The questions addressed by this chapter are the following: First, how serious are the problems faced by state governments in their Medicaid programs? Second, what have the major program trends been in recent years? Third, what are the state governments doing to control the cost of the Medicaid program? Finally, what are the expectations of the state governments with respect to the future of the Medicaid program?

METHODOLOGY

The data for this chapter are derived from the survey of state Medicaid directors conducted during February 1993. The survey utilized a mail questionnaire. The questionnaire contained a total of 80 questions. Seventy-five of the questions were closed-ended, while five questions were open-ended. Some of the questions utilized a five-point scale, while others simply asked the respondents to reply in the affirmative or negative.

Each questionnaire was mailed with a self-addressed, stamped, return envelope. Two separate mailings were utilized. Medicaid directors of 23 states responded to the first mailing. The second mailing was sent to only those who had failed to respond to the first mailing. The second mailing resulted in seven more Medicaid directors responding to the survey. Thus, the total number of respondents to the survey was 30, representing a response rate of 60%.

The 30 state Medicaid directors who responded to the survey represent a diverse group of states. They include large and small states, urban and rural states, industrial and agricultural states. States from all regions of the country are also represented (see Table 2.1).

TABLE 2.1. List of State Respondents and Characteristics of the Medicaid Program

	# of Medicaid Recipients	Total Medicaid Expenditures	State Medicaid Expenditures	Percent of State Budget Consumed by Medicaid
	(Figures are for 1992 — in thousands)			
Alabama	550,000	$ 1,552,990	$ 433,134	17%
Arizona	452,626	$ 1,123,099	$ 372,116	11%
Arkansas	355,000	$ 931,085	$ 233,457	11%
Colorado	243,300	$ 1,030,952	$ 466,340	17%
Florida	1,414,000	$ 3,982,614	$ 1,802,966	16%
Hawaii	97,950	$ 367,326	$ 194,296	5%
Idaho	87,000	$ 243,783	$ 66,456	7%
Illinois	1,346,595	$ 3,670,793	$ 1,879,446	13%
Iowa	296,000	$ 856,316	$ 252,494	8%
Kansas	168,000	$ 542,000	$ 186,000	7%
Kentucky	473,000	$ 1,810,202	$ 521,607	8%
Maryland	460,000	$ 1,786,000	$ 893,000	15%
Massachusetts	620,000	$ 2,800,000	$ 1,400,000	10%
Michigan	1,129,000	$ 3,000,000	$ 1,400,000	18%
Mississippi	490,000	$ 1,100,000	$ 220,000	12%
Missouri	462,000	$ 1,673,735	$ 405,187	17%
Montana	78,057	$ 253,000	$ 62,293	10%
Nebraska	100,000	$ 444,900	$ 137,700	10%
New Hampshire	513,760	$ 332,425	$ 166,213	*
New Mexico	190,524	$ 491,768	$ 128,597	8%
New York	1,500,000	$15,300,000	$ 8,400,000	12%
Nevada	64,000	$ 331,483	$ 161,889	16%
North Dakota	65,659	$ 176,667	$ 40,575	*
Ohio	1,442,300	$ 4,307,723	$ 1,680,012	16%
Oklahoma	360,039	$ 1,003,790	$ 293,709	20%
South Carolina	423,000	$ 1,241,329	$ 168,669	5%
South Dakota	52,000	$ 223,852	$ 60,214	*
Washington	481,000	$ 1,995,707	$ 899,200	13%
Wisconsin	468,800	$ 1,926,300	$ 817,300	12%
Wyoming	55,000	$ 115,720	$ 34,205	11%

* = Did not answer the question.

FINDINGS AND ANALYSIS

Program Characteristics of the Respondent States

The 30 state Medicaid directors who responded to the survey represent a diverse group of states with respect to their Medicaid program characteristics. Large states such as New York, Michigan,

Illinois, Ohio, and Florida serve over a million Medicaid recipients, while small states such as North Dakota, South Dakota, and Nevada have less than 70,000 recipients. Similarly, total Medicaid expenditures (federal and state), as well as state Medicaid expenditures, also vary significantly among the same states. Among the 30 states, the percentage of states' budgets consumed by Medicaid varies from a low of 5% in South Carolina to a high of 20% in Oklahoma. In 20 states, Medicaid expenditures consume 10% or more of the state budget.

Seriousness of Medicaid Problems Faced by the State Governments

There are a number of problems associated with the Medicaid program. The seriousness of the problems varies from state to state. However, as the data in Table 2.2 suggest, some problems are common to almost all states whose Medicaid directors responded to the survey.

TABLE 2.2. Seriousness of Medicaid Problems Faced by State Governments

	Very Serious (1)	Serious (2)	Not Sure (3)	Not Serious (4)	Not Serious At All (5)
Program cost	77%	20%	3%		
Lack of access	10%	55%	3%	28%	3%
Lack of quality care	3%	7%	17%	70%	3%
Federal mandates	30%	53%	7%	10%	
Physician resistance	10%	21%	21%	41%	7%
Increasing number of recipients	33%	53%	10%	3%	
Lack of prenatal care	7%	47%	13%	33%	
The AIDs crisis	7%	33%	27%	30%	3%
Nursing home care	21%	41%	17%	17%	3%
Substance abuse	3%	47%	30%	20%	
"Estate Planning" by elderly	10%	40%	40%	10%	

Note: The sum of the percentages may not equal 100 due to rounding.

One of the biggest problems facing state governments is the dramatically rising cost of the Medicaid program. Ninety-seven percent of the respondents stated that program cost was a serious to very serious problem in their states.

Since its inception, the Medicaid program has experienced dramatic increases in overall cost of the program. The total Medicaid expenditures increased from $5.1 billion in 1970 to $71.3 billion in 1990. The cost to the federal government alone increased from $2.7 billion in 1970 to $40.6 billion in 1990.[5] The program's cost increased by 150% during the 1980s.[6]

State governments have also experienced significant increases in their program costs. The combined cost of the state and local governments for Medicaid increased from $2.3 billion in 1970 to $30.7 billion in 1990.[7] In 1990, Medicaid consumed almost $1 of every $10 of states' tax revenues.[8] Medicaid expenditures, as a percentage of state general expenditures, have grown consistently from less than 3% in 1966 to 14.8% in 1990, with a minor slowdown between 1984 and 1987. According to the National Association of State Budget Officers' projections, state Medicaid spending will reach an average of 17% of state budgets by 1995.[9] The burst of Medicaid spending is contributing to the budget crises of many state governments.

The federal government expects to spend nearly $80 billion on Medicaid in the current fiscal year, while the states plan to spend $60 billion.[10]

A major factor contributing to the dramatically rising cost is the increase in numbers of Medicaid recipients. Of the respondents, 86% viewed the increase in number of program recipients as a very serious or serious problem in their states. The number of Medicaid recipients nationwide increased from 17.6 million in 1972 to 25.3 million in 1990.[11] By 1993, the number of Medicaid recipients had increased to more than 30 million.[12]

Since the dramatic increase in number of recipients to a great extent can be attributed to the program expansion mandated by Congress, it is not too surprising that 83% of the Medicaid directors in the survey viewed federal mandates as a very serious or serious problem facing state governments. Since 1987, Congress has handed down no less than 30 mandates concerning Medicaid eligibility, services, and reimbursement.[13]

Despite the dramatic increase in number of recipients and spending for Medicaid, the program fails to insure millions of poor people who are ineligible to receive Medicaid because they do not fall into one of the eligible categories. Today, Medicaid covers fewer than half of the nation's poor people, mainly because of limits set by state laws regulating eligibility.[14] Ironically, lack of access still remains a major problem. Sixty-five percent of the respondents viewed lack of access as a serious problem facing their states.

Sixty-two percent of the respondents considered the problem of nursing home care as very serious to serious in their states. Over 50% of the respondents stated that lack of prenatal care was a problem in their states, while another 50% cited substance abuse, and Medicaid "estate planning" by the elderly as problems. Forty percent of the respondents viewed the AIDS crisis as a problem, while 30% did not think it was a problem in their states. Some of the states cover the costs of some of the drugs approved by the Food and Drug Administration for treatment of conditions related to AIDS under their Medicaid programs, while others do not.[15] Seventy percent believed that lack of quality care was not a serious problem in their states.

Recent Trends in the State Medicaid Programs

As discussed earlier in this chapter, two major developments occurred in the Medicaid program during the 1980s. One was decentralization of the program and another was federal mandates expanding program coverage, especially to poor women and children. This section examines recent trends in the states' Medicaid programs.

Table 2.3 reports on the trends in states' Medicaid programs. The results are what one would expect, given the two major developments in Medicaid during the 1980s. All respondents reported significant to modest increases in federal mandates. Ninety-three percent of the Medicaid directors in the survey reported significant increases in states' expenditures for Medicaid, while another 3% reported modest increases. As reported in Table 2.1, in 20 of the 30 states responding to the survey, Medicaid consumes at least 10% of the states' total budgets. The proportion of state budgets consumed by Medicaid is increasing. Eighty-three percent also reported a

TABLE 2.3. Recent Trends in States' Medicaid Programs

	Significant increase (1)	Modest increase (2)	Remained the same (3)	Modest decrease (4)	Significant decrease (5)
State Expenditures	93%	3%		3%	
Federal Funds	83%		10%	7%	
Program Access	23%	23%	43%	7%	3%
Quality of Care	7%	40%	53%		
Federal Mandates	67%	33%			
# of recipients	73%	27%			
# of female recipients	62%	35%	3%		
# of AIDS recipients	34%	52%	14%		
# of infant recipients	62%	38%			
# of teenage recipients	36%	54%	11%		
# of elderly recipients	33%	53%	13%		
"Estate Planning" by the elderly	37%	37%	26%		

Note: The sum of the percentages may not equal 100 due to rounding.

significant increase in federal funds. Forty percent believed that there has been a modest increase in the quality of care, while another 7% have seen a significant increase. Forty-six percent of Medicaid directors responding to the survey reported either a significant increase or a modest increase in access to the Medicaid program, while 43% reported that access has remained the same. One of the biggest increases experienced by the state governments was in the number of recipients. Seventy-three percent of Medicaid directors reported significant increases in the number of recipients, while another 27% reported modest increases. When examining the types of recipients, it is clear that Congressional mandates designed to expand coverage for poor women and children have had an impact. The most dramatic increase has been in the number of infants, teenage children, and women. One hundred percent of the Medicaid directors responding to the survey reported that their states had experienced either a significant or a modest increase in the number of infant recipients. Ninety-seven percent reported a modest to significant increase in the number of female recipients. Ninety percent reported a modest to significant increase in the number of teenage recipients.

It is clear that the AIDS crisis has contributed significantly to the problem of program cost. Eighty-six percent of the respondents reported a modest to significant increase in the number of recipients with AIDS. Treatment available for patients with AIDS is very expensive, thus contributing to the program costs.

Eighty-five percent of the respondents reported a modest to significant increase in the number of elderly recipients. Seventy-four percent also reported a modest to significant increase in Medicaid "estate planning" by the elderly in their states. This provides some credibility to the criticism that the Medicaid program is increasingly being used to provide expensive benefits, i.e., nursing home care for middle-class and affluent families. Many families have begun to see Medicaid as a middle-class entitlement program—as a way to preserve the family's life savings and property in the event that one or both parents require high-cost nursing home care.[16] Numerous techniques are utilized for sheltering assets or transferring them to family members as a prelude to getting Medicaid to pay the bill for nursing home care. These include maneuvers such as joint bank accounts; holding property in joint tenancy; investing in irrevocable, nontransferable annuities; and paying family members for services such as shopping and transportation. An army of lawyers and financial advisors counsel affluent Americans on how to shuffle and shelter their elderly family members' assets to qualify for nursing home benefits. Tips on how to shelter one's assets and still qualify for Medicaid are the subject of hot-selling self-help books, financial planning seminars, and adult-education courses.[17] Such maneuvers are called "Medicaid estate planning" and are legal. Nationally, Medicaid has come to pay about 45% of the nation's $53 billion nursing home bill. According to an estimate by the Health Care Financing Administration, Medicaid's nursing home costs will grow two-and-a-half–fold by the year 2000.[18] Despite the "spousal impoverishment" benefit provision passed by Congress in 1988, which substantially raised the amount of income that a spouse could retain before handing the balance over to Medicaid to help defray the cost of a patient's nursing home care, "Medicaid estate planning" is on the rise and is viewed as a serious problem by the states.

State Rationing of Health Care in the Medicaid Program

State governments have responded to the Medicaid program's decentralization, expanded coverage, and rising costs in a variety of ways.[19] Some states have attempted to increase access to health care services for those who are without insurance.[20] This section analyzes how state governments have tried to control the problem of rising costs by rationing Medicaid services.

The advocates of health care rationing argue that we must establish priorities in health services and become more rational in our health care spending. If the United States is serious about containing health care costs, society will have to forego some medical benefits, and patients should not expect to receive all the care they want regardless of the cost.[21] Proponents argue that health care rationing already exists in the actions of the legislatures, insurance companies, hospitals, and physicians.[22] Observers call the existing *de facto* rationing "silent rationing," "under-the-table rationing," "rationing by finance," or "rationing by wallet."[23]

The recent decision by the Clinton administration to grant Oregon's request for a Medicaid waiver is likely to encourage other states to undertake similar measures. Under the Oregon plan,[24] Medicaid will be expanded to cover every person living in poverty within the state. In return, Medicaid services will be rationed. Patients' choices of doctors will be limited, and the state will no longer pay for dozens of procedures deemed too costly or ineffective. The Bush administration had denied Oregon a waiver on the grounds that the plan would violate the Americans with Disabilities Act (ADA) and had asked the state of Oregon to resolve the problem of ADA violations.[25] The Clinton administration was satisfied with Oregon's modifications to the plan.

While most states have not yet gone to the extent of Oregon, many are engaging in some form of rationing of health care services in their Medicaid programs. Table 2.4 reports on how state governments have attempted to ration Medicaid services in their efforts to control costs.

Some states have attempted to reduce the number of Medicaid recipients by tightening eligibility requirements, reducing benefits, and/or by imposing conditions on recipients.[26] One of the ways in which states attempted to control costs in the early 1980s was to reduce the number of Medicaid recipients by reducing eligibility requirements.[27] A significant number of respondents (40%) reported that their states have tightened eligibility requirements for Medicaid

TABLE 2.4. Rationing of Health Care Under State Medicaid Programs

	Yes	No
Eligibility Requirements:		
Tightened eligibility requirements for recipients	40%	60%
Imposed stringent income criteria for eligibility	28%	72%
Eliminated eligibility of persons between ages of 18 and 21	14%	86%
Increased the amount recipients must "spend down" before Medicaid eligibility begins	25%	75%
Benefits:		
Eliminated benefits previously covered by the program	47%	53%
Eliminated/limited coverage for optional services such as dentists, chiropractors, optometrists	50%	50%
Eliminated coverage for weekend hospital admissions	17%	83%
Eliminated payment for in-patient surgery when the surgery could be performed on an out-patient basis	57%	43%
Placed limits on number of visits to doctors, hospitals, etc.	40%	60%
Reduced the number of hospital days covered	27%	73%
Reduced the number of preoperative days covered	33%	67%
Reduced the number of days covered for nursing home care	3%	97%
Reduced utilization of services by recipients	57%	43%
Recipients:		
Required recipients to enroll with an HMO	31%	69%
Restricted recipients' use of providers	55%	45%
Required copayment from recipients for certain services	67%	33%
Established case management program linking Medicaid recipients to solo or group practice physicians	70%	30%
Required elderly recipients to buy long-term care insurance in return for allowing them to retain more of their assets and still be entitled to Medicaid benefits	3%	97%

recipients. Some (25%) have increased the amount recipients must "spend down" before Medicaid eligibility begins. Some states (28%) have imposed stringent income criteria for eligibility, while a few (14%) have eliminated eligibility of persons between the ages of 18 and 21.

Similarly, since the early 1980s, state governments have been active in reducing benefits and imposing other restrictions on their recipients.[28] As the data in Table 2.4 indicate, 50% or more of the Medicaid directors in our survey reported that their states had reduced utilization of services by recipients (57%), eliminated payment for in-patient surgery when the surgery could be performed on an out-patient basis (57%), and eliminated or limited coverage for optional services (50%). A sizable number of respondents said that their states had eliminated benefits previously covered by the program (47%), and placed limits on the number of visits to doctors, hospitals, etc. (40%). Some have reduced the number of preoperative days covered (33%), hospital days covered (27%), or eliminated coverage for weekend hospital admissions (17%).

In addition, many states have imposed various conditions on the recipients. A large majority of states in the survey indicated that they required copayments from recipients for certain services (67%), while others restricted recipients' use of providers (55%). Some states required recipients to enroll with an HMO (31%). A large majority of state respondents (70%) have established case management programs linking Medicaid recipients to solo or group practice physicians. Such programs have become very common.[29]

Some states require Medicaid patients to participate in managed care programs. For example, New York, Massachusetts, and Oregon have enacted legislation authorizing a rapid expansion of managed care for almost all Medicaid recipients. California and Maryland have recently moved in the same direction, requiring managed care for all recipients who fail to specify that they have ongoing relationships with particular providers. Maryland's plan limits recipients to relationships with physicians who will act as gatekeepers.[30] Many advocates of expanded managed care claim that it can save money and increase access at the same time. However, a number of studies of managed care plans have demonstrated that to a large extent such plans have failed to improve access for the recipients.[31]

It is clear from the above discussion that rationing of Medicaid services has become common among many states. Options such as tightening eligibility standards, reducing benefits, or imposing conditions on the recipients are attractive options for the state governments since state agencies are the ones who make such decisions, and they have the machinery to calculate the amount of savings that can be generated. However, critics argue that such methods are most likely to adversely affect low-income patients.[32] Opponents of rationing plans such as Oregon's argue that the main target of rationing is the poor—mainly women and children who make up most of the Medicaid population.[33] Attempts to control costs during the last five years have reduced access to care for the poor and uninsured, and future attempts to control costs may compound the access problem further.[34] Some do not view HMOs as an answer to these problems. They argue that the promise of HMOs for Medicaid remains unfulfilled, especially in a voluntary environment.[35] However, some recent empirical analyses suggest that state Medicaid policies designed to contain costs by limiting utilization appear to affect neither access nor utilization.[36]

New State Initiatives in the Medicaid Programs

State governments have also attempted to control Medicaid costs by undertaking new initiatives with respect to health care providers, bulk rate purchasing of certain equipment and services, engaging in negotiated or competitively bid fixed price arrangements,[37] hospital rate-settings,[38] and the use of Medicaid waivers.[39] Table 2.5 reports states' initiatives in these areas.

A large number of state respondents have cut prices paid to providers (63%) and locked out providers who have been found to provide too many unnecessary services or poor quality of care (57%). A majority of states have imposed a provider tax[40] on hospitals and other health care providers (63%). Such a provider tax was designed to get more matching funds out of the federal government. Congress, in 1991, moved to curb this practice by imposing certain restrictions on the states. These restrictions include: (1) in order to receive federal matching funds, such taxes must be broad-based, imposed uniformly, and include all members of a class such as all in-patient hospitals, all physicians, or all HMOs; (2) these taxes

TABLE 2.5. New Initiatives in the State Medicaid Programs

	Yes	No
Health Care Providers:		
Cut prices paid to the providers	63%	37%
"Locked out" providers who have been found to provide too many unnecessary services or poor quality of care	57%	43%
Imposed an extra tax (provider tax) on hospitals and other health care providers	63%	37%
Bulk Rate Purchases:		
Purchased, in bulk, durable medical equipment, lab tests, X-ray services, etc.	20%	80%
Used bulk purchase arrangement for various goods such as eyeglasses, hearing aids, etc.	41%	59%
Medicaid Waivers:		
Used Medicaid waivers for home and community-based services for the elderly	93%	7%
Used Medicaid waivers for home and community-based services for the mentally ill	47%	53%
Used Medicaid waivers for home and community-based services for the physically disabled	93%	7%
Fixed Price Arrangements:		
Engaged in negotiated fixed price arrangement with health care providers	43%	57%
Engaged in competitively bid fixed price arrangement with health care providers	23%	77%
Engaged in negotiated and/or competitively bid fixed price arrangement with hospitals	17%	83%
Engaged in negotiated and/or competitively bid fixed price arrangement with nursing homes	7%	93%
Engaged in negotiated and/or competitively bid fixed price arrangement with physicians	7%	93%
Hospital Rate-Setting:		
Utilized mandatory rate-setting for hospital payments	57%	43%
Encouraged voluntary compliance by hospitals with the results of the state review process	39%	61%
Cost-based rate-setting program	92%	8%
Revenue-based rate-setting program	8%	92%

cannot make up more than 25% of a state's share of Medicaid; and (3) such taxes cannot contain a "hold harmless" provision which guarantees that health care providers will have the tax they paid returned to them.[41]

A majority of the states (57%) in the survey indicated that they use mandatory rate-setting for hospital payment, while some (39%)

encourage voluntary compliance by hospitals with the state review process. States which use the rate-setting program tend to rely largely on cost-based rate-setting programs (92%) and not on revenue-based programs (8%). Such rate-setting programs have been in practice since the early 1980s. The results of rate-setting programs on cost-containment have been mixed.[42] Many state governments, in the late 1980s, revised their rate-setting formulas to reduce payments to providers. This, in turn, has led health care providers to file lawsuits against state governments for what they consider inadequate reimbursements. States have lost many cases, thereby forcing them to pay millions of dollars more in reimbursements to health care providers.[43]

Forty-one percent of the respondents indicated that they use a bulk rate purchase arrangement for various goods such as eyeglasses, hearing aids, etc., while a few states (21%) engaged in the practice of bulk rate purchase of durable medical equipment, lab tests, and X-ray services.

Forty-three percent of states engaged in a negotiated fixed price arrangement, while 23% engaged in a competitively bid fixed price arrangement with health care providers. However, the practice is not very common with respect to physicians and nursing homes.

Section 2176 of the 1981 OBRA allows states to seek waivers from the Department of Health and Human Services for a variety of home and community-based services provided to certain individuals such as the elderly, physically disabled, developmentally disabled, and the mentally ill who would otherwise receive more costly nursing home care.[44] Waivers also provide states with the means to secure additional federal funding for services that otherwise would have been funded entirely through state revenues. Our survey indicated that such practices are very popular with state governments. An overwhelming majority (93%) of the states in the survey indicated that they have used Medicaid waivers for home and community-based services for the elderly and the physically disabled, while 47% indicated that they had used the waivers for the mentally ill.

New Programs Initiated by State Governments

State governments have also created new programs aimed at reducing the costs of their Medicaid programs. Table 2.6 provides some data on new programs established by the state governments. Almost all of the states who responded to the survey indicated that they had established family planning/child care programs (90%) and prenatal care programs (87%). A large majority of states had established teenage pregnancy prevention programs (70%), AIDS education programs (67%), and substance abuse prevention programs (57%). A sizable number of states (41%) had established antismoking campaigns, while others had established catastrophic insurance programs (33%). The data indicate that the state governments are trying to address some of the cost problems by emphasizing prevention and/or primary care with specific emphases on women and the young.

TABLE 2.6. New Programs Initiated by State Governments

	Yes	No
Pre-natal care program	87%	13%
Substance abuse prevention program	57%	43%
Teenage pregnancy prevention program	70%	30%
AIDS education program	67%	33%
Catastrophic insurance program	33%	67%
Family planning/child care program	90%	10%
Anti-smoking program or campaign	41%	59%

Expectations About the Future of the Medicaid Programs

What are the perceptions and expectations of the state Medicaid directors about the future of the Medicaid programs in their states? Table 2.7 provides some insights.

Despite all the measures taken to contain Medicaid costs, almost all of the Medicaid directors (97%) responding to the survey indicated that they expect modest to significant increases in state expenditures, as well as modest to significant increases in the number of recipients. An overwhelming majority (86%) of the states' Medicaid directors expect to receive modest to significant increases in federal funds. A majority (57%) expect to see modest to significant increases in federal mandates. Ironically, a majority also expect

TABLE 2.7. Expectations About the Future of the Medicaid Programs

	Significant increase (1)	Modest increase (2)	Remained the same (3)	Modest decrease (4)	Significant decrease (5)
State expenditures	64%	33%			3%
Federal funds	53%	33%	7%	7%	
Program access	28%	28%	34%	10%	
Quality of care	13%	40%	47%		
Federal mandates	21%	36%	32%	7%	4%
# of recipients	37%	60%		3%	
Rationing	12%	36%	48%	4%	
Managed care	60%	33%	7%		
Managed competition	43%	36%	21%		

Note: The sum of the percentages may not equal 100 due to rounding.

access to their programs (56%), as well as quality of care (53%) to increase in the future.

Forty-eight percent of the respondents expect modest to significant increases in rationing of Medicaid services. An overwhelming majority of respondents also see modest to significant increases in managed care and managed competition.

CONCLUSION

The decentralization of the Medicaid program by the Reagan Administration in the early 1980s gave state governments greater flexibility to experiment with new approaches in delivering health care to the poor. The subsequent program expansion through congressional mandates significantly increased the number of recipients plus program costs. Concerned with the dramatically rising cost of the program that is consuming a larger and larger portion of state budgets, state governments have used the Medicaid program in innovative ways to respond to the access and health care financing issues. Some have experimented with service delivery, payment reforms, and outreach programs. These approaches have included rationing of Medicaid services, increased use of Medicaid waivers for home or community-based services, fixed price arrangements with health care providers, hospital rate-setting, and bulk-rate purchase of certain equipment and services. More emphasis has also been placed on case management and managed care. Many states have established new programs designed to provide preventive and primary care.

The results of these experiments have been mixed. While a few have been successful in containing specific costs, the overall cost of the program continues to rise both at the federal and state levels. Rationing in the Medicaid program leads to concerns about reduced access and limited choices. The same concern is raised with managed care programs. Reduction in payments to physicians has often made them more reluctant to accept Medicaid patients. Hospital rate-setting programs, in general, have not been very successful.

Increased micromanagement of the Medicaid program by the federal government through Congressional mandates has created additional problems for states. State governments' abilities to fund their programs at the current service levels are severely tested. The problem is compounded by a growing case load, declining revenue, and balanced budget requirements. States are being sued by hospitals and other health care providers over reimbursement rates. In a majority of cases states have been the loser. The crisis of escalating cost is not likely to be resolved until the problems of long-term care, reimbursement levels, and the uninsured are addressed in one form or another.

All the new state experiments and innovations have failed to produce any consensus on how best to contain costs. These experiments have offered many different models of cost containment, but none is satisfactory to all parties. It is clear that the program cannot continue on its current course given stagnant or declining resources on the one hand and pressure to provide coverage to more people on the other hand. Additional ad-hoc, stopgap fixes are likely to produce more dissatisfaction with the program among various groups such as policy makers, health care providers, program administrators and advocacy groups. Perhaps the best news is that the Clinton administration's revised health care plan, designed to overhaul the health care system, would incorporate Medicaid recipients and other low-income people into the same network of doctors, hospitals and private insurance companies that serves more affluent people. This is promising because it would end the two-tier health care system we currently have—one for the rich and another for the poor.

NOTES

1. D. Altman, "Health Care for the Poor," *The Annals of the American Academy of Political and Social Sciences,* vol. 468 (July 1983): 112–113.

2. J. Kosterlitz, "Middle-Class Medicaid," *National Journal* (November 9, 1991): 2728–2731.

3. P.R. Lee and C.L. Estes, "New Federalism and Health Policy," *The Annals of the American Academy of Political and Social Sciences,* vol. 468 (July 1983): 100.

4. For a detailed analysis of the evolution of health care policy and its implications for federalism, see F.J. Thompson, "New Federalism and Health Care Policy: States and the Old Questions," *Journal of Health Politics, Policy and Law,* Vol. 11, No. 4, Tenth Anniversary Issue (1986): 647–669; also, see P.R. Lee and C.L. Estes, "New Federalism and Health Policy," pp. 88–102.

5. K.R. Levit et al., "National Health Expenditures, 1990," *Health Care Financing Review,* Vol. 13, No. 1, Fall, 1991, pp. 41, 51 and 52 (29–54).

6. M. Specter, "Medicaid's Crazy Quilt of Care," *The Washington Post National Weekly Edition,* August 26–September 1, 1991, p. 33.

7. K.R. Levit et al., "National Health Expenditures, 1990," pp. 51 and 52.

8. R.J. Samuelson, "Medicaid Monster," *The Washington Post National Weekly Edition,* May 2–26, 1991, p. 29.

9. E.J. Dubin, "Medicaid Reform: Major Trends and Issues," *Intergovernmental Perspective,* Vol. 18, No. 2, Spring, 1992, p. 5 (5–9).

10. R. Pear, "Clinton Considers Stopping Medicaid Under Health Plan," *The New York Times,* March 29, 1993, p. Al. c 2, East United States Edition.

11. K.R. Levit et al., "National Health Expenditures, 1990," p. 41.

12. R. Pear, "Clinton Considers Stopping Medicaid Under Health Plan," *The New York Times,* March 29, 1993, p. A1. c2, East United States Edition.

13. J. Horvath, "Medicaid: Successes, Failures, and Prospects," *Intergovernmental Perspective,* Vol. 18, No. 2, Spring, 1992, p. 13 (12–24, 29).

14. R. Pear, "Clinton Considers Stopping Medicaid Under Health Plan," *The New York Times,* March 29, 1993, p. A1. c2, East United States Edition.

15. "Survey of State Medicaid Coverage of AIDS-Related Drugs," prepared by Intergovernmental Health Policy Project, The George Washington University for the Health Care Financing Administration, U.S. Department of Health and Human Services, Washington, DC, June 1990.

16. D.P. Baker, "Squeezing through the Loophole in the Medicaid Law," *The Washington Post National Weekly Edition,* March 2–8, 1992, p. 34.

17. Melinda Beck et al., "Planning to be Poor," *Newsweek,* November 30, 1992, p. 66 (66–67).

18. J. Kosterlitz, "Middle-Class Medicaid," *National Journal,* November 9, 1991, p. 2729 (2728–2732).

19. For a brief state-by-state analysis, see Intergovernmental Health Policy Project, The George Washington University, *Major Changes in State Medicaid Programs, 1990,* Health Care Financing Administration, U.S. Department of Health and Human Services, August, 1991.

20. For analysis of how some states are trying to provide coverage to the uninsured, see U.S. General Accounting Office, *Access to Health Care: States Respond to Growing Crisis,* Washington, DC: Government Printing Office, June, 1992.

21. H.J. Aaron and W.B. Schwartz, *The Painful Prescription: Rationing Hospital Care,* Washington, DC: The Brookings Institution, 1984.

22. P.T. Menzel, *Strong Medicine: The Ethical Rationing of Health Care,* New York: Oxford University Press, 1990.

23. V. Cohn, "Rationing Medical Care," *The Washington Post National Weekly Edition,* August 13–19, 1990, p. 11.

24. To understand the history of Oregon's rationing plan, see J. Kitzhaber, "A Healthier Approach to Health Care," *Issues in Science and Technology,* Vol. 7, (Winter 1990–1991): 59–65; T. Egan, "Oregon Shakes Up Pioneering Health Plan for the Poor," *The New York Times,* February 22, 1991, p. 11; P. O'Neill, "Oregon's Health Care Rationing Plan Causing Fight," *Health Career News,* September 12, 1990, pp. 17–21; and M. Beck and N. Joseph, "Not Enough for All: Oregon's Experiments with Rationing Health Care," *Newsweek,* May 14, 1990, pp. 53–54.

25. J.P. Shapiro, "To Ration or Not To Ration?" *U.S. News and World Report,* August 10, 1992, p. 24.

26. D.E. Altman and D.H. Morgan, "The Role of State and Local Governments in Health," *Health Affairs,* Vol. 2, No. 4, Winter 1983, p. 26.

27. R.B. Bovbjerg and J. Holahan, *Medicaid in the Reagan Era: Federal Policy and State Choices,* Washington, DC: The Urban Institute Press, 1982, pp. 30–31.

28. K. Johnson, "Major Surgery for Ailing Medicaid Program," *U.S. News and World Report,* October 17, 1983, pp. 91–93.

29. R.G. Kern and S.R. Windham with P. Griswold, *Medicaid and Other Experiments in State Health Policy,* Washington, DC: American Enterprise Institute for Public Policy Research, 1986, p. 54.

30. M. Melden, "Medicaid Recipients: The Forgotten Element in Medicaid Reform," *Intergovernmental Perspective,* Vol. 18, No. 2, Spring, 1992, p. 15 (15–17).

31. R. Kotelchuck, "Medicaid Managed Care: A Mixed Review" *Health/PAC Bulletin,* Vol. 22, No. 3, Fall, 1992, pp. 4–11; D.A. Freund et al., "Evaluation of the Medicaid Competition Demonstrations," *Health Care Financing Review,* Vol. 11, Winter, 1989, p. 81; and M.D. Anderson and P.D. Fox, "Lessons Learned from Medicaid Managed Care Approached," *Health Affairs,* Vol. 71, Spring, 1987, p. 80.

32. D. Altman, "Health Care for the Poor," p. 115.

33. J. Kosterlitz, "Rationing Health Care," *National Journal,* June 30, 1990, pp. 1590–1595; and J.W. Fossett et al., "Medicaid and Access to Child Health Care in Chicago," *Journal of Health Politics, Policy, and Law,* Vol. 17, No. 2 Summer, 1992, pp. 273–298.

34. L. Wagner, "Access for All People," *Modern Health Care,* July 28, 1989, p. 26 (26–34).

35. J.L. Buchanan et al., "HMOs for Medicaid: The Road to Financial Independence is Often Poorly Paved," *Journal of Health Politics, Policy, and Law,* Vol. 17, No. 1, Spring, 1992, p. 94 (71–96).

36. C.J. Barrilleaux and M.E. Miller, "Decisions Without Consequences: Cost Control and Access in State Medicaid Programs," *Journal of Health Politics, Policy, and Law,* Vol. 17, No. 1, Spring, 1992, p. 110 (97–118).

37. J. Holahan, "The Impact of Alternative Hospital Payment Systems on Medicaid Costs," *Inquiry,* Vol. 25, No. 4, Winter, 1988, pp. 519–520; R.J. Vogel, "An Analysis of Structural Incentives in the Arizona Health Care Cost-Containment System," *Health Care Financing Review,* Vol. 5, No. 4, Summer, 1984, pp. 13–22; and J.S. McCombs and J.B. Christianson, "Applying Competitive Bidding to Health Care," *Journal of Health Politics, Policy and Law,* Vol. 12, No. 4, Winter, 1987, pp. 703–712.

38. J. Holahan, "The Impact of Alternative Hospital Payment Systems on Medicaid Costs"; and D.A. Crozier, "State Rate-Setting: A Status Report," *Health Care Financing Review,* Vol. 4, No. 2, Summer, 1982, pp. 66–83.

39. S.S. Laudicina and B. Burwell, "Profile of Medicaid Home and Community-Based Care Waivers, 1985: Findings of a National Survey," *Journal of Health Politics, Policy, and Law,* Vol. 13, No. 3, Fall, 1988, pp. 528–529.

40. For a history of this controversial practice, see J.P. Shapiro, "How States Cook the Books," *U.S. News and World Report,* July 29, 1991, pp. 24–25; W. Tucker, "A Leak in Medicaid," *Forbes,* July 8, 1991, pp. 46–48; R. Pear, "U.S. Moves to Curb Medicaid Payments for Many States," *The New York Times,* September 11, 1991, p. 1; H. Dellios, "Hospitals Hit Deal on Medicaid," *Chicago Tribune,* November 23, 1991, p. 5.

41. T. Hudson, "States Scramble for Solutions Under New Medicaid Law," *Hospitals,* Vol. 66, No. 11, June 5, 1992, p. 52 (52–56)

42. For a discussion of pros and cons of the rate-setting programs, see C. Coelen and D. Sullivan, "An Analysis of the Effects of Prospective Reimbursement Programs on Hospital Expenditures," *Health Care Financing Review,* Winter 1981; J. Holahan, "The Impact of Alternative Hospital Payment Systems on Medicaid Costs"; S.A. Mitchell, "Issues, Evidence, and the Policymaker's Care," *Health Affairs,* Vol. 1, No. 3 (Summer, 1982, pp. 84-98); D. Rosenbloom, "New Ways to Keep Old Promises in Health Care," *Health Affairs,* Vol. 2, No. 4, Winter, 1983, pp. 41–55; and F.A. Sloan, "Reviews: An Economist," *Health Affairs,* Vol. 1, No. 3 Summer 1982, pp. 113–118.

43. R. Pear, "Suits Forces U.S. and States to Pay More for Medicaid," *The New York Times,* October 29, 1991, p. 1; D. Durda, "Number of Lawsuits Belies Complexities Involved in Such Filing," *Modern Health Care,* Vol. 21, No. 8, February 25, 1991, pp. 31–32; and R. Pear, "Ruling May Lead to Big Rise in States' Medicaid Costs," *The New York Times,* July 5, 1990, p. 8.

44. S.S. Laudicina and B. Burwell, "Profile of Medicaid Home and Community-Based Care Waivers, 1985: Findings of a National Survey," *Journal of Health Politics, Policy, and Law,* Vol. 13, No. 3, Fall, 1988, pp. 528–529.

Chapter 3

Primary Prevention with the Poor: Structural Conflicts Between the Health and Welfare Systems

Patricia A. Nolan

The special nature of prevention services creates significant problems in delivering these services to the poor American society. These problems arise from the close relationship between poverty and the antecedents of disease: poor nutrition, poor sanitation, crowding, and lack of health care services. The welfare model of delivery services to the poor exacerbates the difficulties of providing prevention services to them. Dependency is rewarded, and a bare minimum of services is provided because of cost and eligibility constraints. Prevention services are intended to be provided to well persons and may not meet the definition of "medically needed" which is frequently a requirement of health care programs in the welfare mode. In addition, prevention services are low technology services, poorly compensated to the provider.

The State of Arizona has made an effort to use a cost-controlled health maintenance model to deliver health services to the very poor. The program, the Arizona Health Care Cost Containment System (AHCCCS), is a modification of Title XIX program allowed under the Medicaid waiver provisions. The results of this program have not been salutary for many of the people it was planned to serve. Administrative procedures, especially those designed to control

This chapter was originally published in *Journal of Health & Social Policy*, Vol. 1(1) 1989.

43

costs and determine eligibility, have been so costly themselves that public dollars are diverted from health care services to administration. Some of the most productive prevention strategies have not been supported through the AHCCCS program. Meanwhile, the poor who are ineligible for, or not enrolled in, AHCCCS are receiving even fewer health services than before.

Theoretically, enrolling the poor in an HMO-model health care provider should increase the access to preventive medicine services. There are structural barriers in the Arizona version of the Medicaid program which significantly reduce the provision of these services to the poor. These are: (1) the enrollment process, (2) the concept of "medically-required" services, (3) short-term eligibility and mandatory reenrollment, (4) automatic assignment without regard to the current source of care, (5) significant financial disincentives to providers who actively seek out those in need of prevention services, and (6) the exclusion of family planning services from the program.

The enrollment process of a welfare program in the United States is designed to assure that only those who meet strict income and asset criteria receive the services of the program. The process starts from the assumption that a person is not entitled to the services. Demonstrating entitlement is time-consuming, demeaning, and difficult, not likely to be undertaken just to get a periodic check-up. Some enrollees in federal welfare programs are automatically entitled to benefits; for example, those receiving Aid to Families with Dependent Children and Supplemental Security Income. These beneficiaries are assigned to provider groups and notified of their enrollments, based upon successful completion of an equally rigorous eligibility process.

Starting with the assumption that a person should not receive the services helps create a second barrier to preventive services. Both the provider and the client operate from a perspective that the client is receiving something for nothing. Since Medicaid is "intended" to provide only "medically-required services," prevention services can be pictured as luxuries by both providers and recipients. The message is clearly communicated that health care is for only the "really sick."

The requirement for frequent reenrollment creates a barrier to continuity of care. The AHCCCS program adds another wrinkle through the provider bidding process: The provider may change because a provider group drops out or fails in the bidding process. This is especially problematic in management of chronic illness, and in the provision of common forms of preventive medicine, such as prenatal care and childhood immunizations. Cultural barriers are more significant when there are no long-term patient-provider relationships. Communication of important prevention and health promotion information is difficult if there is no shared vocabulary. Changing providers can represent so much effort that the client stops seeking care.

The AHCCCS program automatically assigns new enrollees to a plan based upon the bid process, not upon the current source of care. Thus, a pregnant patient receiving prenatal care from a physician when her husband loses his job, may automatically be assigned to a new provider when she becomes AHCCCS enrolled, even though her current physician is an AHCCCS provider. Patients who do not reenroll promptly may be assigned to new providers when they do reenroll.

Preventive medicine is not the practice model followed by every physician. Prevention is not the lifestyle model of many people, including those receiving services through Title XIX. Years of experience in the delivery of prevention services in the public sector and through neighborhood health centers have shown that it is essential to actively seek out clients to promote participation in prevention. Enrolling people in a managed-care program does not assure adoption of prevention behaviors, or even contact with the provider unless severe illness occurs. The financial incentives for active prevention efforts are diluted if the client does not come for services, especially if the client subsequently loses eligibility or is assigned to another group. Among the poor, communication with health care professionals may not seem benign. Going to the doctor may be associated with severe illness or the threat of death, rather than with learning how to live a healthier life. The absence of financial incentives for providing specific outreach and primary prevention services works against the success of the capitation system at the core of the AHCCCS program: the enrollees of this program are not schooled in the practice of seeking prevention services.

The most startling example of these financial disincentives is the decision by the legislature to exclude an important prevention program altogether: family planning services have not been provided. This decision resulted in fragmentation of care to women, since routine gynecologic care and family planning services are combined for most of us. It also results in expensive duplication of such basic health care services as pelvic examinations. In 1988, the legislature remedied this omission, but allowed plans to opt out of providing services for religious reasons. This mixed message on the legitimacy of family planning services may also perpetuate duplication.[1]

Yet, theoretically, "integrating prevention and medical care is less expensive, more convenient, more administratively efficient, and has more community impact than keeping them separated," as Roemer has contended.[2] The model of the Arizona Health Care Cost Containment System fails in preventive care, not because of the capitation model, nor because the prevention and therapeutic services are to be integrated, but because the emphasis remains the welfare pattern. As long as keeping people off the roles and limiting services to those "medically needed" is the primary emphasis of publicly-supported health care programs, prevention will not be successfully provided through them.

The AHCCCS program has not lived up to its billing in a number of ways, some related to the bidding and administrative concepts built in by the legislature. The delivery of health care through enrollment of recipients with a provider group responsible for primary care and the determination of need for specialty care can effectively deliver both preventive and therapeutic health services. AHCCCS is saddled with unwieldy eligibility and enrollment procedures and with disincentives for outreach and specific prevention services built in by the legislature to control costs. As long as our intention is to restrict health care services to the poor, we will be unable to achieve the benefits of current knowledge about the prevention of disease and the promotion of health.

NOTES

1. ARS 36-2901 et seq as amended, 1988, and rules adopted subsequent to statute.

2. Roemer, M. *An Introduction to the U.S. Health Care System.* New York: Springer Publishing, 1986.

BIBLIOGRAPHY

Addy, L., and Anderson, R., "A Framework for the Study of Access to Medical Care." In *Issues in Health Services,* S.J. Williams, ed. New York: John Wiley and Sons, 1980.

Lopes, P. (ed.). "Health Care for the Notch Group: How Do We Assure Accessibility to Services?" Health Systems Agency of Southeastern Arizona, 1989.

Chapter 4

The Health Consequences of Economic Recessions

Loring Jones

Unemployment has been demonstrated to be a stressful life event with severe health consequences. In fact it is suggested that the evidence to link unemployment with morbidity and mortality is so strong that it should be necessary to include a warning slip from the Surgeon General with every pink slip that unemployment is hazardous to your health (Brown, 1983). Unemployment reduces the resources available for health care and creates stressful situations for laid-off workers and families. Stress has long been recognized as a major contributor to the development of a variety of physical and mental illnesses (Brenner, 1977).

Social workers practicing in health care settings may be in the front line of encountering problems that are associated with economic turndowns. Researchers have found that despite the loss of health insurance that follows a lost job the need for health care may increase (Buss and Redburn, 1983; Kasl and Cobb, 1978; Linn, Sandifer, and Stein, 1985). The increase in the need for health care occurs not only because of an upsurge in physiological symptoms, but because for many of the unemployed psychological distress may be expressed in terms of physical symptoms (Kasl and Cobb, 1978; Gore, 1979; Krystal et al., 1983; Rayman, 1982).

Depression has been found to be a significant problem among the unemployed. Many of the symptoms of depression are exhibited in

This chapter was originally published in *Journal of Health & Social Policy*, Vol. 3(2) 1991.

physical complaints such as exhaustion, sleep disturbance, loss of appetite, and generalized aches and pains. Social workers in health care settings may be in the front line of the social welfare system during economic turndowns because working class populations perceive social services and mental health services offered in other agencies as stigmatizing and thus to be avoided. They are more likely to express physical complaints than psychological complaints (Buss and Redburn, 1983; Liem and Liem, 1978; Rayman, 1982). Therefore it is important that social workers in health care be aware of the needs of this population.

The 1981–1982 recession brought social workers into contact with unemployed working class individuals who may never have had previous contact with the social service system. In many instances these individuals lacked sophistication in knowledge of available services and how to use them. On the other hand social workers may not know how to meet this group's needs. This chapter reviews the literature on the relationship between unemployment and health for the purpose of identifying how macroeconomic change affects health. Social workers need to gain an understanding of the linkage between psychosocial and economic functioning.

THE RESEARCH EVIDENCE
ON THE HEALTH EFFECTS OF JOB LOSS

The most influential types of research on the relationship between unemployment and health in terms of influencing decision makers have been those using large scale aggregate data. The most important of this type of work has been the widely quoted work of Brenner (1978, 1984), who correlated an increasing unemployment rate and other changes in labor market activity with the increase of various health ills such as cardiovascular ills, cirrhosis diseases, suicide, infant mortality, homicide, motor vehicle accidents, child abuse, and psychiatric admissions to name a few. Brenner finds that in the first year of an economic downturn there is a sharp increase in psychological symptoms that is measured in increasing suicide rates, and psychiatric hospital admission increases. Two to three years after the onset of the recession, which may occur in the peak of the recovery, problems with mortality and morbidity become apparent because of the lag inherent in pathological processes associated with life events (Holmes and Rahe, 1967). Brenner (1984) and others who have done similar types of research have been criticized because of the ecological fallacy. It cannot be said that any job loser is suffering difficulty since these researchers are comparing rates. These studies leave open the possibility that job loss has a detrimental impact on others rather than just the job loser. Even persons who maintain continuous employment during periods of recession may also find their health adversely affected. Another criticism of this type of research is that it fails to specify the intervening variables between economic change and the deterioration of health status. Also the cross-sectional nature of the data does not allow one to address the direction of change in health status.

An adjunct to the aggregate data research has been the individual level studies done with small samples of workers in specific situations such as plant shutdowns. The longitudinal nature of these studies with their panel designs has addressed the issue of causation and has identified some of the intervening variables that account for adverse outcomes (Buss and Redburn, 1983; Catalano, Dooley, and Rook, 1987; Eisenberg and Lazarsfeld, 1938; Gore, 1979; Iverson and Sabroe, 1988; Iverson, 1987; Liem and Rayman, 1982; Linn, Sandifer, and Stein, 1985; Margolis and Farran, 1983; McKenna and McCewen, 1987; Parnes and King, 1977; Perrucci et al., 1985; Rayman, 1982; Warr and Jackson, 1985).

These studies have demonstrated that employment status predicts health status. The unemployed reported more physical complaints, took more medication, had higher blood pressure, made more emergency room visits, and had more hospital admissions than employed workers. These findings have held true even in the studies that have controlled for selection bias. Selection bias or the "uncovering hypothesis" postulates an alternate explanation that employers discharge people who are in marginal physical or mental health. Because of their conditions these workers find it harder to find reemployment, and are more likely to manifest difficulties when out of work (Schwefel et al., 1984; Dooley and Catalano, 1984). Studies that have used baselines for health prior to notification of shutdown, or have attempted to control for reason of discharge, still find that health deteriorates after job loss even among those in prior good health. These effects on health status have been found to extend to family members of the job loser.

Children are dependent on the economic success of their parents. When the economy turns sour they are caught in the middle. Not only do their parents have fewer resources, but children find less support from social programs than they have found in the past. Ten million children were affected by their parents' unemployment in the 1981–1982 recession (Rayman, 1987). During that period 3 million children fell below the poverty line (Edelman, 1986). These children are at risk because for most children including those with mild medical problems, family socioeconomic status is the best single predictor of children's health status, and the level of psycho-social development (Butler, Starfield, and Stenmark, 1982).

One example of the risks that children face in economic downturns is that the infant mortality rate increases at a lag of up to two years which suggests damage occurs both in utero and in the environment after birth (Brenner, 1978, 1984). The increase may be due to having less resources for prenatal and pediatric care. Nutrition may decline and mothers and families are under increased stress.

Children experience the effect of economic deprivation through changes in family consumption patterns. Children are the group most affected by the weakness in the public and private insurance systems. In 1984 children made up 25% of all Americans under 65, but they comprise one-third of all uninsured persons (Children's Defense Fund, 1986). A consistent finding in the literature is that the unemployed defer most health care. One example of this reduction in health care can be seen with dentistry which is seen by many unemployed families as a luxury. Only emergency dental care is likely to be sought (Johnson and Abramovitch, 1985). Lack of preventative care contributes to more severe problems later.

A number of studies have indicated that children experience similar reactions to unemployment as do their parents. These studies indicate that children of the unemployed report more somatic complaints, are at greater risk to incur illness, have disabilities of longer duration, experience more sleep disturbances, have more eating disorders, and have more accidents than children of employed workers (Madge, 1983; Margolis and Farran, 1981; Buss and Redburn, 1983; Rayman, 1987).

Two clear indicators of the health risks to children emerge in the evidence that links unemployment with the increasing incidence of child abuse, with some evidence to indicate that the severity of that abuse increases during joblessness (Galdston, 1965; Gil, 1971; Justice and Duncan, 1978; Light, 1973; Miraga, 1982; Madge, 1983; Steinberg, Catalano, and Dooley, 1981). The other indicator of risk is the report by Garfinkel, Froese, and Hood (1982), that children with unemployed parents were twice as likely to be admitted to pediatric emergency rooms for suicide attempts.

A major deficit in the research is the lack of attention given to women's unemployment (Marshall, 1984). Research prior to this point has largely been in studies of the effects of white male unemployment. This deficit in regard to women is a reflection of outmoded beliefs about the place of women and their earnings. However, a number of studies have associated employment with better health in women, and women's job loss with the development of the health difficulties similar to those that men develop (Dooley and Catalano, 1984; Hibbard and Pope, 1985; Kessler, House, and Turner, 1987; Parry, 1986; Verbrugge, 1983). Verbrugge (1983) found unemployed women have more short-term health problems and fewer long-term problems than unemployed men. It is not surprising that women are responsive to the negative aspects of job loss with more women finding work to be a necessity. The studies of male unemployment indicate wives and children experience health difficulties similar to the males, but perhaps with a time lag (Liem and Rayman, 1982).

Longitudinal studies that have followed the unemployed for at least two years have found that health complaints increased in the first year and stabilized or decreased in the second year (Catalano, Dooley, and Rook, 1987; Iverson and Sabroe, 1988; Buss and Redburn, 1983; Gore, 1979; Iverson, 1987; Kasl, Gore, and Cobb, 1975). Kasl and colleagues (1975), who monitored the health status of workers in two plant closings, found physical complaints were highest in the phase of anticipation before the shutdown. Their findings suggest health damage begins before job loss and is related to increased insecurity. A study of Danish shipyard workers found a similar pattern of complaints. A control group of shipyard workers who were not facing layoff also showed elevated symptoms during the anticipation phase. The researchers interpreted their findings to mean the controls were aware of the shutdown and were fearful for their own jobs (Iverson and Sabroe, 1988). It follows that plant shutdowns or recessions may increase problems by generating insecurity among the larger group of people who keep their jobs.

The exclusive focus on the unemployed during periods of downturns may neglect other potential risks. There may be increased stress, insecurity, and guilt among people who keep their jobs. There may be competitive relationships among those still-employed staffs, and at the same time resentment toward these "survivors" by the unemployed (Brockner, Davy, and Carter, 1985). Workers may feel stressed by heavy work loads as they take up the slack of laid-off workers. There is also the possibility of less attention being paid to health and safety factors by firms operating under financial pressures.

INTERVENING VARIABLES BETWEEN ECONOMIC CHANGE AND HEALTH STATUS

The most obvious and direct route to difficulty is financial. The main tie into the health system for most Americans comes through the health insurance acquired on the job, which is then lost when unemployment occurs. According to a Presidential commission staffed by Reagan appointees, the number of Americans not covered by private insurance or public health programs reached 53 million Americans during the 1981–1982 recession (Brown, 1983). Despite the subsequent recovery, the number of Americans without any kind of health insurance stands at 37 million. Many of those job losers who went back to work did so at lower wages and without benefits such as health insurance (Bluestone and Harrison, 1982; Kessler, House, and Turner, 1987). Families can also suffer from reduced resources that lead to a decline in nutrition and housing quality that adversely affects health.

The unemployed defer most health care and wait until situations reach crisis proportions before seeking treatment. This delay complicates treatment and adds to the cost of intervention. Most Americans approach health care as a discretionary expense. In the absence of public and private insurance, and in the presence of financial pressures on the household budget, most Americans will delay all but emergency care (Madonia, 1983). Even then the choices of treatment used might not be the most desirable. In the emergency room, the treatment is one-shot treatment instead of continuity care that might more successfully treat difficulties. The result is that problems become more serious and difficult to treat.

Unemployment has been found to be a stressful life event. Many researchers see an important psychosocial route to health difficulty is the chronic physiological arousal that involves excessive coping demands leading to a state of exhaustion, and a suppression of the immune system (Brenner, 1978; Brenner and Mooney, 1983; Buss and Redburn, 1983; Eyer, 1977; Liem and Liem, 1978). Researchers in psychosomatic medicine have indicated that various personality and stress conditions are contributing factors in the development of specific diseases such as the coronary illness, identified by Brenner (1984) as particular risks during economic turndowns.

Unemployment has been found to be disruptive of social networks which may then deprive a person of a potential reservoir of social support. Social support has been identified as a critical buffer of the health consequences of adverse life events (Atkinson, Liem, and Liem, 1987; Aiken and Ferman, 1966; Bolton and Oakley, 1987; Buss and Redburn, 1983; Gore, 1979; Iverson and Sabroe, 1988; Kasl, Gore, and Cobb, 1975; Kessler, House, and Turner, 1987; Linn, Sandifer, and Stein, 1985; Warr and Jackson, 1985). These studies find that the unsupported exhibit more illness complaints and depression than the supported. Social network support has also been identified as a crucial aid in the return to work (Vinokur and Caplan, 1987).

Immoderate habits may develop which are attempts to alleviate stress but in themselves contribute to health difficulties. A number of studies have noted an increase in alcohol consumption, drug usage, smoking, eating disorders, and sleep disturbances (Brenner, 1978 and 1984; Brenner and Mooney, 1983; Burke, 1984; Johnson and Abramovitch, 1985; Kessler, House, and Turner, 1987; Liem and Rayman, 1982; Perrucci et al., 1985; Schwefel et al., 1984; Sunley and Sheek, 1986).

At the macro level there are a number of ways recession can contribute to ill health even among those who keep their jobs. A recession creates a situation at the macro level where there are fewer resources available to improve the standard of living, such as investments in health care services, public health services, or decent housing. All of these lead to an increase in health problems in the general population.

A number of trends in the economy such as the phenomena of "deindustrialization" suggest that for many, health risks will not disappear with reemployment. Individuals may be forced to accept reduced wages and benefits through "give backs." Underemployment in terms of pay, benefits, skills, and working conditions are becoming pervasive features of the economy, and the effects of these on psychosocial and health functioning need to be investigated. Workers may be demoralized, perhaps degraded, and on a path of downward mobility. These families have fewer resources to devote to health care (Bluestone and Harrison, 1982; Iatrides, 1988; Kessler, House, and Turner, 1987). If downward mobility does occur one can invoke the considerable body of literature that links declining social status to a variety of health ills.

The passage of an "early warning" plant notification law by Congress would put additional responsibility on social workers in the area of unemployment because there would now be an opportunity to anticipate increased stress in the community. The advance notice provision of the new law might help create a lobby to enable social agencies to go into plants which anticipate layoffs and provide services. The provision of such services might be built into the unemployment insurance program. In the absence of such social policies there are some immediate strategies that social workers can adopt to meet an upsurge in need.

STRATEGIES FOR SOCIAL WORK INTERVENTION

Social work intervention with the unemployed should occur in three areas. First, efforts are needed to maintain or replace jobs. Second, resources are needed to help maintain a continuity of health care. Finally, psychosocial supports are needed to help the unemployed cope with the negative psychosocial aspects of unemployment that are a threat to health.

Efforts to Maintain or Replace Jobs

It is recognized that in a less than full employment economy, there are limits to a social work role in regard to unemployment because joblessness is primarily an economic event. Unemployment does have a psychosocial component that is within the purview of social work. Economic policies have an enormous impact in the lives of social work clients. Therefore social workers need to be involved in the shaping of these policies as researchers, analysts, and advocates (Sherraden, 1985). Hardly an economic policy arises that does not affect health status. One social work role is to engage in fact finding on the health aspects of unemployment in order to provide data for decision makers. At least some policy makers may be reluctant to continue to accept higher levels of unemployment as the norm if they understood that the cost added to a recession is the treatment of health problems. At times of macroeconomic change, social workers in health care could collect data on such health indicators as hospital admission rates, emergency room utilization, and mortality and morbidity rates to name a few. These statistics would lend weight to advocacy arguments.

Provision of Resources

Aggressive outreach is needed to reach a population unaccustomed to using the social service system. This reluctant population needs help in securing benefits in order to ensure a continuity of health care. Individuals and families need to be reached before their problems develop into crises proportions and treatment becomes greatly complicated. The provision of resources may reduce the stress in families which left unattended may lead to additional problems.

Health care social workers may be the "tripwire" for psychosocial problems in any economic downturn because of the great number of health problems among the unemployed, and their propensity to somatically express psychological problems. It would seem important that health care workers assess the occurrence of a recent major stressor, such as unemployment, that might trigger the seeking of health care. Linn, Sandifer, and Stein (1985) cite data to back their claim that physicians often do not know the patient's employment status.

Provision of Psychosocial Services

The evidence is convincing that the health effects are greatest in the first year of unemployment and are likely to stabilize thereafter.

Even in the first year symptoms are likely to be concentrated in the early phases of job loss. This pattern of effects suggests a service delivery strategy based upon the life events literature. This literature suggests that preparation reduces the worst effects of adverse life events. In situations of anticipated closings a preventative strategy can be taken that educates families about what is to be expected in regard to the psychosocial and financial aspects of unemployment by reducing anxiety and uncertainty, and helping people become aware of services that they might need in the future. Such information can be dispensed through a group work format, pamphlet, or use of the media. The assumption is that the knowledge provided reduces the population that would need more intensive services at a later date.

Populations that have been identified as having particular difficulties with reemployment can be targeted with more intensive services over the long term. These groups include older males, minorities, women, and particularly women with children (Flaim and Sehgal, 1985; Moen, 1979).

Group work self-help efforts are the most consistently suggested interventions for the unemployed worker (Briar, 1983; Buss and Redburn, 1983; Fedrau, 1984; Kasl and Cobb, 1978; Keiselbach and Svensson, 1987; Madonia, 1983; Shore, 1984). There is some evidence to indicate that self-help efforts are the preferred way for this group to receive services (Shelton, 1985).

Shore (1984), a social worker who practices in the San Francisco area, describes a program whereby social agencies provided outreach workers to go to such sites as union halls. These workers provided information and referral, and helped train peer counselors who conducted the actual groups. Outreach and group self-help programs find considerable support in the practice literature on unemployment because the unemployed are often unaccustomed to using social services, and may feel stigmatized by seeking those services. Outreach and the group approach are assumed to break through the reluctance to use services and allay the features of stigma associated with help seeking (Rayman, 1982).

Buss and Redburn (1983) speculate that one factor that accounted for stabilization of symptoms in the second year of their Youngstown study was that a large number of community-based organizations had proliferated to help people cope with the shutdown. The groups came from traditional social action organizations, social agencies, churches, and unions. These types of group interventions were seen as an aid in helping to combat isolation, empower workers, provide a sense of usefulness, legitimize services, and in giving the workers a means to secure reemployment. These groups were also possible reservoirs of social support. The importance of social support in preventing and reducing illness, and effecting a more rapid recovery, has significant support in the literature (Ell, 1984).

The ecological perspective has increased social workers' awareness that problems that people bring agencies are seldom one-dimensional and have many facets. The most effective contribution a social worker can make to practice with the unemployed is not to separate concrete needs from underlying psychological or physical health problems (Shore, 1984). In dealing with the unemployed it should be recognized that many families do not attribute their difficulties to unemployment. Problems such as marital conflict, child behavioral problems, school difficulties, or substance abuse may be outcomes of unemployment, and not the results of individual family dynamics. Almost all the longitudinal studies indicate that high levels of symptoms expressed during job loss will at least begin to recede with reemployment. Efforts to help a return to work may be the most effective type of treatment for many unemployed. Just as health care social workers are knowledgeable of how to make referrals to the mental health or child welfare systems, they should have knowledge of how clients would use employment and training services in their communities.

It has been shown that one way to cope with the impact of life events is to help people reappraise the meaning of the event. The evidence suggests that those who successfully cope with job losses are those who define unemployment as an opportunity and challenge (McKenna and McCewen, 1987; Little, 1976). Helping individuals plan for new employment as early as possible after the notification of layoff would be a preventative strategy.

CONCLUDING COMMENT

The erosion of support in federal programs will place the unemployed at risk in the next recession. Many people have been encouraged to think that government participation in the economy makes them immune to experiencing the worst effects of unemployment (Schlozman and Verba, 1978). This assumption is mistaken. The risks for the unemployed may be greater in the next recession because we will enter the downturn with high numbers of people already out of work, and those who do lose their jobs will find less support than they would have found at earlier times. Such a situation is difficult for the social service system because line workers are in danger of burnout from high caseloads. There was a documented upsurge in referrals from the private to public medical facilities, and an upsurge in the first-time users of public health services in Detroit, during the last recession (Gold, 1984). Private agencies have the difficulty of facing a population that may not have a way to pay for services. One way to relieve stress on both the health care system and families that are still on the horizon is a National Health Insurance scheme that would break the bonds between access to health care and participation in the labor market. Until such a time recessions and plant closings will present major public health problems.

REFERENCES

Aiken, M., and Ferman, L.A. (1966). Job mobility and social integration of the displaced worker. *Social Problems, 14*(1), 48–56.

Atkinson, T., Liem, R., and Liem, J. (1987). Unemployment: Implications for social support. *Journal of Health and Social Behavior, 27*(12), 317–331.

Bluestone, D., and Harrison, B. (1982). *The Deindustrialization of America.* New York: Basic Books.

Bolton, W., and Oakley, K. (1987). A longitudinal study of social support and depression in unemployed men. *Psychological Medicine, 17*(2), 453–460.

Brenner, M.H. (1977). Personal stability and economic security. *Social Policy, 8*(1), 2–5.

Brenner, M.H. (1978). Health and the national economy: Commentary and general principles. In L.A. Ferman and J. Gordus (eds.), *Mental Health and the Economy.* Kalamazoo, MI: Upjohn Institute, 63–85.

Brenner, M.H. (June 1984). Estimating the effects of economic change on national health and social well-being. A study prepared for use of the Subcommittee on Economic Goals and Intergovernmental Policy, Joint Economic Committee, U.S. Congress. Washington, DC: U.S. Government printing office.

Brenner, M.H., and Mooney, A. (1983). Unemployment and health in a context of social change. *Social Science and Medicine, 14,* 1125–1138.

Briar, K.H. (1983). Unemployment: Toward a social work agenda, *Social Work, 28*(3), 211–216.

Brockner, J., Davy, J., and Carter, C. (1985). Layoffs, self-esteem, and survivors guilt: Motivational, affective, and attitudinal consequences. *Organizational Behavior and Human Decision Making Processes, 36,* 229–242.

Brown, B. (1983). The impact of political and economic changes upon mental health. *American Journal of Orthopsychiatry, 53*(4), 583–592.

Burke, R.B. (1984). The closing of Canadian Admiral: Correlates of individual well-being 16 months after shutdown. *Psychological Reports, 55*(1), 91–98.

Buss, T., and Redburn, F.S. (1983). *Mass Unemployment, Plant Closings and Mental Health.* Beverly Hills: Sage studies in community mental health.

Butler, J., Starfield, S., and Stenmark, S. (1982). Child health policy. In H. Stevenson and A. Siegel (eds.), *Child Development Research and Social Policy.* University of Chicago Press.

Catalano, R., Dooley, D., and Rook, K. (1987). A test of reciprocal risk between undesirable economic and non-economic life events. *American Journal of Community Psychology, 15*(5), 633–651.

Children's Defense Fund (1986). *Children's Defense Budget: An Analysis of F.Y. 1987 Federal Budget and Children.* Washington, DC.

Dooley, D., and Catalano, R. (1984). Why the economy predicts help seeking behavior. *Journal of Health and Social Behavior, 25,* 160–175.

Edelman, M.W. (1986). *Families in Peril: An Agenda for Social Change.* Cambridge, MA: Harvard University Press.

Ell, K. (1984). Social networks, social support, and health status: A review. *Social Service Review, 58,* 133–149.

Eyer, J. (1977). Prosperity as a cause of death. *International Journal of Health Services, 7*(1), 125–150.

Fedrau, R.H. (1984). Easing the worker's transition from job loss to unemployment. *Monthly Labor Review, 107*(5), 38–40.

Flaim, P., and Sehgal, P. (1985). Displaced workers, of 1979–1983: How well did they fare? *Monthly Labor Review, 108*(7), 3–16.

Galdston, R. (1965). Observations of children who have been physically abused by parents. *American Journal of Psychiatry, 122,* 440–443.

Garfinkel, B., Froese, A., and Hood, A. (1982). Suicide attempts in children. *American Journal of Psychiatry, 139,* 1257–1261.

Gil, D. (1971). Violence against children. *Journal of Marriage and the Family, 33*(4), 637–657.

Gold, S. (1984). Prepared statement before the Select Committee on Children, Youth, and Families. House of Representatives, 98th Congress, Second session, Detroit, MI.

Gore, S. (1979). The effects of social support in moderating the health consequences of unemployment. *Journal of Health and Social Behavior, 19*(2), 157–165.

Hibbard, J., and Pope, C. (1985). Employment status, employment characteristics and women's health. *Women's Health, 10*(1), 59–77.

Holmes, T.H., and Rahe, R.H. (1967). The social readjustment rating scale. *Psychosomatic Medicine, 11,* 213–218.

Iatrides, D. (1988). New social deficit: Neoconservatism's policy of social under-development. *Social Work, 33*(1), 1–17.

Iverson, L. (1987). Some health effects of the closing of a Danish shipyard in a three year followup. In P. Pederson and P.O. Lund (eds.), *Unemployment Theory, Policy, and Structure.* Berlin, GDR: DeGruyter, 305–320.

Iverson, L., and Sabroe, S. (1988). Psychological well-being among the unemployed after a company shutdown. *Journal of Social Issues, 44*(4), 141–152.

Johnson, L., and Abramovitch, R. (1985). *Unemployed Fathers: Parenting in a Changing Labor Market.* Toronto: Social Planning Council.

Justice, B., and Duncan, D. (1978). Child abuse as a work related problem. *Corrective and Social Psychiatry, 23*(1), 53–55.

Kasl, S.V., and Cobb, S. (1978). Some mental consequences of plant closing and job loss. In L.A. Ferman and J. Gordus (eds.), *Mental Health and the Economy.* Kalamazoo, MI: UpJohn Institute, 255–295.

Kasl, S.V., Gore, S., and Cobb, S. (1975). The experience of loss of job: Reported changes in health, symptoms, and illness behavior. *Psychosomatic Medicine, 37*(2), 106–122.

Keiselbach, T., and Svensson, P. (September 1987). Health policy and development in Europe in response to economic instability. Paper presented at the International Conference of Social Welfare, Rome, Italy.

Kessler, R., House, J., and Turner, B. (1987). Unemployment and health in a community sample. *Journal of Health and Social Behavior, 28*(1), 51–59.

Krystal, E., Sackett, M.T., Thompson, S., and Cantoni, L. (1983). Serving the unemployed. *Social Casework, 64*(2), 67-72.

Lazarsfeld, P., and Eisenberg, P. (1938). The psychological effects of unemployment. *Psychological Bulletin, 35*(6), 358–392.

Liem, H.C., and Liem, J.H. (1978). Social support and stress: Some general issues and their application to the problem of unemployment. In L.A. Ferman and J. Gordus (eds.), *Mental Health and the Economy.* Kalamazoo, MI: UpJohn Institute, 347–377.

Liem, R., and Rayman, P. (1982). Health and social cost of unemployment. *American Psychologist, 37*(1), 1116–1123.

Light, R.J. (1973). Abused and neglected children in America: A study of alternatives. *Harvard Educational Review, 43*(4), 556–598.

Linn, M., Sandifer, R., and Stein, S. (1985). The effects of unemployment on mental and physical health. *American Journal of Public Health, 75*(5), 502–506.

Little, C.B. (1976). Technical-professional middle class adaptability to personal crisis. *The Sociological Quarterly, 1*(2), 262–274.

Madge, N. (1983). Unemployment and its effect on children. *Journal of Child Psychology and Psychiatry, 24*(2), 311–319.

Madonia, J.H. (1983). The trauma of unemployment and its consequences. *Social Casework, 64*(8), 482–488.

Margolis, L.H., and Farran, D.C. (1981). Helping families of unemployed workers. *North Carolina Medical Journal, 42*(2), 849–850.

Margolis, L.H., and Farran, D.C. (1983). Unemployment and children. *International Journal of Mental Health, 13*(2), 107–124.

Marshall, C. (1984). On the sociology of women's unemployment: Its neglect and significance. *Sociological Review, 32*(2), 234–259.

McKenna, S., and McCewen, J. (1987). Employment and health. In D. Fryer and P. Ullah (eds.), *Unemployed People: Social and Psychological Perspectives.* Pittsburgh: Open University Press.

Miraga, T. (1982). Unemployment's youngest victims. *Education Week, 2,* 1–15.

Moen, P. (1979). Family impacts of 1975 recession. *Journal of Marriage and the Family, 41*(3), 561–572.

Parnes, H.S., and King, R. (1977). Middle-aged job losers. *Industrial Gerontology, 4,* 77–95.

Parry, G. (1986). Paid employment, life events social support, and mental health in working class mothers. *Journal of Health and Social Behavior, 27*(2), 193–208.

Perrucci, C., Perrucci, R., Tarq, H., and Tarq, D. (1985). The impact of plant closings. *Research in the Sociology of Work, 3,* 231–260.

Rayman, P. (1982). The world of not working: An evaluation of the urban social service response to unemployment. *Journal of Health and Human Resource Administration, 1,* 320–333.

Rayman, P. (1987). Unemployment and family life: The meaning for children. In P. Voyandoff and L. Majka (eds.), *Families in Economic Distress: Coping Strategies and Social Policy.* Beverly Hills, CA: Sage Publications.

Schlozman, K.L., and Verba, S. (1978). The new unemployment: Does it hurt? *Public Policy, 26*(3), 333–353.

Schwefel, D., Jurgen, J., Potthoff, P., and Hechler, A. (1984). Unemployment and mental health: Perspectives for the Federal Republic of Germany. *International Journal of Mental Health, 13*(1), 25–30.

Shelton, B. (1985). The social and psychological impact of unemployment. *Journal of Employment Counseling, 22*(3), 18–22.

Shore, L. (1984). The Fremont experience: A counseling program for dislocated workers. *International Journal of Mental Health, 13*(1–2), 154–168.

Sherraden, M.W. (1985). Chronic unemployment: A social work perspective. *Social Work, 30*(5), 403–408.

Steinberg, L.D., Catalano, P., and Dooley, D. (1981). Economic antecedents of child abuse and neglect. *Child Development, 52,* 975–985.

Sunley, R., and Sheek, G.W. (1986). *Serving the Unemployed and Their Families.* Milwaukee, WI: Family Service Association.

Verbrugge, L.M. (1983). Multiple roles and physical health of women and men. *Journal of Health and Social Behavior, 24*(1), 16–30.

Vinokur, A., and Caplan, R. (1987). Attitudes and social support: Determinant of job seeking behavior and well-being among the unemployed. *Journal of Applied Social Psychology, 17*(12), 1007–1024.

Warr, P., and Jackson, P. (1985). Factors influencing the psychological impact of prolonged unemployment and reemployment. *Psychological Medicine, 15*(4), 795–807.

Chapter 5

Health and Poverty in Canada

Donald R. Leslie

INTRODUCTION

This chapter presents an overview of the Canadian health care system and explores some relevant issues in the area of health and poverty. The geographical proximity of Canada to the United States has long made it appropriate to compare and contrast the two health care approaches of these countries. This chapter will review some of the more salient similarities and differences in terms of overall health impacts, particularly in relationship to issues of income and poverty. As well, the two systems will be contrasted with regard to cost effectiveness and administrative efficiency.

The contention that the Canadian health care system is one of the "best in the world" will be examined in regard to health and the impact of poverty. Areas of successful health intervention will be highlighted, but the myth of universal health coverage as a health panacea is challenged by the author. In addition, some of the future trends in Canadian and North American society will be examined with respect to their implications for both the health care system and overall health impacts for the poor and economically marginalized individuals.

HISTORY OF THE CANADIAN HEALTH CARE SYSTEM

Similar to most social welfare programs based upon attempts to implement national social policy, the Canadian health care system did not emerge as a complete entity, but rather evolved over time. Its evolution moved forward through a blend of both provincial and federal initiatives. This blending of provincial and federal jurisdictions has its roots in *The British North America Act* of 1867 and the resultant programs and approaches have been markedly influenced by the British "cradle to grave" social welfare ideology. However, the development of national health policies in Canada were also influenced significantly by regional values, beliefs, and circumstances as well as the influence of the French Canadian culture. The view from outside of Canada, as a nation with a standardized and universal health care system, is only partially accurate. While there is a relatively coherent social policy approach to the provision of health care across the nation, the major responsibilities for health care administration and implementation rest with Canada's provinces and territories. Even today, there are marked differences in basic coverage, accessibility, and direct service health programs from province to province.

It is fair to say that the core principles included in national health policy do, however, ensure that the system implemented in each part of the country does accomplish the basic provision of health care for all Canadian residents. Indeed, five principles must be adhered to by all jurisdictions in order to meet the criteria for participation in the federal cost sharing of health services. The five principles of *universality, accessibility, comprehensiveness, portability,* and *public administration* are enshrined as basic requirements in all provincial and territorial health delivery systems (Badgley and Wolfe, 1992; Clarke, 1990; Kunitz, 1992; Nair, Karim, and Nyers, 1992; National Council of Welfare, 1990; Vayda and Deber, 1992). Thus, while the federal government of Canada has no clear constitutional jurisdiction in this area, it has evolved a significant role in the standardization of health services through its constitutional jurisdiction over general taxation revenues and their subsequent disbursement.

The principle of *universality* ensures that all Canadians are entitled to basic health care services irrespective of their social economic status. The only eligibility requirement for inclusion in each of these health service plans is that of legal residency. No provincial or territorial health service system is allowed to exclude any individual from coverage with respect to employment status, social situation, prior health history, or preexisting conditions. Through the criterion surrounding this principle, Canada ensures coverage for all its people without actually operating a national health service. While some anomalies such as provision of services to aboriginal peoples, worker's compensation, and specialized service delivery programs do exist, such programs must at least meet the criteria for implementation of this and the other four principles.

The principles of *accessibility* and *portability* can be seen as corollaries to the principle of *universality.* The criteria and standards derived from these principles ensure access to health services regardless of personal circumstance and ensure that reciprocal agreements between jurisdictions exist such that individuals moving from province to province experience no lapse in their health coverage.

The principle of *comprehensiveness* leads to criteria for services covered as implemented by each jurisdiction. The specific range of services covered vary somewhat from province to province, but they must ensure the existence of basic health services. At a minimum these plans must ensure unimpeded access to and coverage for physician services, hospitalization, public health services, and most surgical procedures. Provincial plans vary in terms of the inclusion of pharmacological services, adaptive devices, and paramedical services (e.g., chiropractic, physiotherapy, dental, etc.). Despite minor anomalies in the provincial and territorial plans, the system provides all residents with basic comprehensive health services.

The principle of *public administration* has thus far meant that the basic comprehensive health services available to all residents of Canada have remained securely under government control. Criteria derived from this principle, while replicated from province to province, have functionally produced a single-payer process for basic comprehensive health care. In addition, provisions for funding of hospital services have ensured the predominance of not-for-profit facilities and ancillary support programs. However, implementation of these five principles throughout the various jurisdictional plans has fostered and protected the entrepreneurial and autonomous functioning of physicians. In addition, the system leaves room for and has encouraged the development of the continued role of private or for-profit insurance companies in the provision of additional or extended benefits such as drug plans, dental insurance, eye care, and enhanced semiprivate or private hospital coverage plans.

As mentioned, the current Canadian health care system has evolved over time and through the policy initiatives of different jurisdictions. The idea of a universal health care system was proposed as early as 1919 and the ideological foundations for such a system were researched and written about by Leonard Marsh in Quebec in the 1930s (Badgley and Wolfe, 1992; Bellamy and Irving, 1995; Turner, 1995). However, most historians credit the birth of Medicare in Canada to initiatives taken in the province of Saskatchewan. In this province, a hospital services plan was established in 1947 and was expanded to a more comprehensive health services plan during the 1950s and early 1960s. The acceptance of this Medicare system had popular support from its beginning with speculation that experiences of The Great Depression and "Dust Bowl" of the 1930s helped to dislocate the ideal of personal effort in relation to economic security. Indeed, the bulk of western prairie farmers and those dependent upon the agro-economy found themselves victims of the weather and the larger economy irrespective of their hard work. However, the acceptance by the medical profession did not come as easily, with Saskatchewan experiencing the first ever physicians' strike in 1962 (Clarke, 1990; Evans, 1993; Kunitz, 1992). Despite this shaky beginning, current surveys of physicians in this province and in Canada in general, show relatively high levels of support for a universal, comprehensive health care system.

The federal government began to take national initiative in health care policy and passed legislation establishing public health insurance in 1966 with expansions and modifications to this legislation occurring in 1972 and 1977. The current legislation, *The Canada Health Act*, was passed in 1984 and ensured that medical care would be financed out of the public purse. This act also prohibited the practice of so-called "extra billing" for services covered in the basic comprehensive plan. Implementation of this standard in the province of Ontario once again resulted in a physicians' strike. To date, the operationalization of a Canadian health care policy remains a delicate balancing act among federal and provincial jurisdictions along with provincial and national medical associations under the watchful scrutiny of Canadian consumers.

COMPARISONS OF CANADIAN AND U.S. SYSTEMS

Both Canadians and Americans see their health services as being the "best in the world." Without question, the resources in the United States devoted to medical technology, education, and research certainly make it a leader in the field. However, medical training, availability of technology, and development of medical techniques are shared across national borders. In fact, the United States and Canada share a common process for accreditation of physician training (Evans, 1993; Vayda and Deber, 1992). Certification for physicians and paramedical professionals is usually no more difficult between Canada and the United States than among the various U.S. states. In large part, the skills, knowledge, and routine technologies provided to individuals seeking health services in either country do not vary significantly.

There is some validity to the Canadian assertion of having the best health care system. Indeed, many countries have researched and studied the Canadian system because of its international reputation (Badgley and Wolfe, 1992; Beatty, 1993). This reputation has been based in part upon Canada's ability to provide its residents with universal, comprehensive, publicly funded health care despite its small population and immense geography. In truth, comparisons of U.S. and Canadian health services are akin to comparing apples and oranges. While both are edible, seed-bearing fruits, their tastes and peculiarities are worlds apart.

No nation's health care system can be understood in isolation from the values, beliefs, and cultural context of its peoples. Indeed, what allows for a positive health care program is the goodness of fit between the national psyche and the health service system as viewed by the general population. Thus, any comparison among systems must be done with a view to enhancing knowledge and understanding of one's own approach rather than for the purpose of importing system dynamics from another approach.

In the popular press and public rhetoric of the United States, one of the most striking views of the Canadian health care system is that it represents "socialized medicine." This very terminology conjures images of health service rationing and enforced physician selection. The reality could not be further from the truth. In order to contrast the two systems in a meaningful way, it is important to examine a number of operational elements within both systems. These elements include: physician practices, hospitalization, consumer coverage, administration, and funding.

Ironically, American fears of socialized medicine often revolve around issues of physician selection, and autonomous decision making between doctors and patients. In Canada, the system allows for individuals to select any physicians of their choice, and all basic services are available based upon physician-patient choice. The bulk of physicians operate as private practitioners with high levels of professional autonomy. In contrast, the advent of MHOs, PPOs, and other forms of medical practice organization in the United States have functionally reduced an individual's right to physician selection and often impinge upon physician autonomy in the area of treatment choices.

Similarly, views of long waiting lines and rationing of services spring to mind when Americans think about Canada's socialized medicine. In fact, as health care needs have outstripped health care resources in both countries, waiting lists and service delays have come into existence. In the Canadian system, availability of services is moderated by medical need, while U.S. consumers find availability moderated, at least in part, by insurance company regulations and the ultimate ability to pay for services. From an outside view, it appears that the working poor are the most disadvantaged in the U.S. system, while in Canada, the wealthy must suffer the indignity of not being able to jump to the front of the line simply because of their financial resources. In reality, neither the American nor Canadian system deserve the label of "socialized medicine" in this regard.

Both the U.S. and Canadian health care systems provide a broad base of access to hospitalization; however, major differences exist in terms of coverage and accessibility. The United States draws heavily upon a charities model approach in providing hospital services to the uninsured, and access to particular hospitals and facilities within hospitals may be determined by private insurance and ability to pay. The Canadian system provides coverage through the universal health insurance system and while access to private or semiprivate rooms may be dictated through access to private insurance, the same facilities are often allocated upon the basis of medical need and physician decision irrespective of ability to pay. Organizationally, the systems differ in that many U.S. hospitals and medical facilities function as private, profit-making corporations, while the vast majority of Canadian facilities are nonprofit organizations operating under locally elected, autonomous boards.

As already noted, universal health care coverage in Canada provides all residents with equal access to a comprehensive range of health services. Although private insurance still provides a range of extended benefits, Canadians, in general, are secure in their access to health services regardless of their social and/or financial situations. In large part, this removes anxieties with regard to preexisting conditions, medical catastrophes, and issues of concern for medical benefits when employment is lost or changed, unlike the situation for employees in the United States. The advent of Medicaid and Medicare in the United States has resulted in protection for many U.S. residents, but large gaps in coverage still exist, particularly for the working poor (Summer, 1994). In addition, employees with corporate health benefits must think seriously about portability of these benefits when considering employment changes or when affected by the seemingly ever present "downsizings."

Consumer surveys in the United States and Canada perennially show significant differences in levels of perceived satisfaction with each country's health care systems. Terris (1990) quotes a Harris poll as showing 10% of Americans think their system works "pretty well" as compared to 56% of Canadians holding the same view of their own system. The same poll indicated 61% of Americans would trade the U.S. health care system for the Canadian system, while only 3% of Canadians would trade for the U.S. model.

The impacts in the areas of administration and funding can be viewed together. U.S. health services are funded diversely through charitable dollars, a wide range of government funding programs, private insurance revenues, and private corporate enterprises. This diverse funding process leads to complex administration procedures adding cost to the overall system (Beatty, 1993; Evans, 1993; Nair, Karim, and Nyers, 1992). Even though the Canadian system incorporates provincial and territorial jurisdictions, the strong federal presence in standards-setting creates a process analogous to a single-payer system. This single-payer system results in less administration and a somewhat tighter cost control process (Pollack, 1993). This difference in complexity of administration is often cited as the reason for overall cost differences between the two systems. For example, in 1960, prior to Canada's implementation of universal health care, both Canada and the United States devoted slightly over 5% of GDP to health care. Recent estimates report the U.S. health care system as absorbing 12.2% of the GDP, while the Canadian system absorbs 9.2% of its GDP (Nair, Karim, and Nyers, 1992).

Canadians are rightfully proud of their health care system's ability to provide universal, comprehensive health care for almost one-third less the cost of the U.S. system. The price paid for this system is not, as speculated by many Americans, "socialized medicine," but rather is closer to socialized funding, or more appropriately, overt public funding (Evans, 1993). When viewed in terms of government support, the Canadian system represents one of the most expensive systems in the world. However, it must be remembered that this refers to public support for health care rather than the overall costs of providing health care to its population (Madore, 1993). At the same time, gross outcome measures such as longevity (U.S. males 71.6 years, and females, 78.6 years, versus Canadian males, 73.7 years, and females, 80.6 years; and infant mortality per 100,000—United States ten, and Canada seven) show the systems to be comparable on these measures or if anything favoring Canada slightly (Nair, Karim, and Nyers, 1992). By way of example, Table 5.1 presents information summarizing death rates for selected causes, and reinforces the view that the universal, comprehensive health care system in Canada shows certain benefits not achieved under the U.S. model.

While the above discussions make it clear that the application of the label "socialism" is not appropriate to either system, it is apparent that the two systems are underpinned by different social values and political structures. Historically, Canadians have traditionally embraced a broader range of collectivist values as opposed to the rugged individualism underlying many U.S. policies. This emphasis on collectivist values opened the door for Canadian social welfare and health care policies to embrace an overall institutional view of service provision. The individualistic perspective of U.S. society

TABLE 5.1. Age-Standardized Death Rates per 100,000 Population for Selected Causes for Men

Causes	Canada, 1989	U.S.A., 1988
Infectious diseases	5.8	14.2
Cancer	259.6	245.7
Cardiovascular diseases	381.8	456.1
Respiratory diseases	88.3	95.3
Digestive diseases	35.2	38.3
Liver diseases	13.8	16.8

Note: Adapted from "Health Care and Health Status: A Canada-United States Statistical Comparison," by C. Nair, R. Karim, and C. Nyers, 1992, *Health Report*, Vol. 4 No. 2, p. 181.

has resulted in an adherence to a more residual approach to social and health policies. In summary, the Canadian and U.S. health care systems share many similarities, have some striking differences, but appear to be consistent with the underlying core values espoused by each nation.

HEALTH OUTCOMES AND POVERTY

Issues related to assessing the overall health and well-being of a nation's people are extremely complex. Certainly, the nature and availability of health services and the service delivery system are assumed to have major impacts on health maintenance. However, even within this narrow scope, arguments rage over the relative importance and impact of prevention programs, service delivery systems are criticized for being illness reactive, and issues of personal responsibility abound. Viewed in the larger context, issues of general nutrition, sanitation, water quality, exercise, and lifestyle cannot be discounted as variables affecting general health (Wilkins, 1995). In addition, even broader categories of economic growth, employment stability, general social welfare programs, and societal health values cannot be ignored as contexts influencing overall health patterns.

Along with the myriad of complex variables affecting health, there is disagreement with and difficulty in defining and obtaining appropriate indicators or measures of health. At one level, there are numerous difficulties with the validity and interpretation of gross statistical measures such as mortality rates, longevity, and health surveys (Badgley and Wolfe, 1992; Blackburn, 1991; Clarke, 1990; Lepore, 1994; Power, Manor, and Fox, 1991; Roberge, Berthelot, and Wolfson, 1995b; Zambrana, 1988). The tendency to quote such measures as correlates to narrow variable clusters such as existing health service programs is fraught with difficulty. As well, current trends in gross statistical outcomes are often utilized without respect to historical fluctuations or directions. For example, the trend in increased longevity since the establishment of the Canadian universal health care system shows a marked improvement from 1956 (70 years) to 1995 (77 years). Such figures demonstrate an improvement which clearly achieves both statistical and practical significance. However, the current trend ignores a preexisting trend which showed a change in longevity figures from 1926 (58 years) to 1956 (70 years), which predates the existence of a universal health care system (Badgley and Wolfe, 1992). One way of combating this fallacy of interpretation is to examine other possible variable sets which theoretically may also be correlated with the overall outcome measures (Anderson and Armstead, 1995). For example, one of the major predictors for general health is that of the impact of poverty or resource distribution. Undeniably, the categorization of poverty or income variables is every bit as complex as general health and well-being itself, but nonetheless, exploring this relationship in conjunction with health can be instructive (Adler et al., 1994; Schiller, 1989).

Figures shown in Table 5.2 illustrate the assumed association between income levels and health as measured by overall longevity (National Council of Welfare, 1990). These data show the impact of categorizing by neighborhood income levels. In particular, life expectancy for males shows a clear deterioration in association with income level, while the impact on longevity for females is less pronounced (poorest, 79.1 years, to richest, 80.9 years).

Similarly, Table 5.3 provides a comparison of male Health Status Index scores by three levels of household income and age catego-

TABLE 5.2. Life Expectancy of Canadian Males by Neighborhood Income, 1986

Type of Neighborhood	Years of Life at Birth
Poorest	70.4
Second Poorest	73.5
Middle	74.4
Second Richest	75.3
Richest	76.1

Note: Adapted from *Health, Health Care and Medicare,* p. 7, by The National Council of Welfare, Canada, 1990. Ottawa: Minister of Supply and Services.

TABLE 5.3. Health Status Index Scores for Men in Canada by Income Levels

Age	Income Level		
	High	Middle	Low
25-34	96%	95%	92%
35-44	95%	95%	92%
45-54	94%	92%	87%
55-64	92%	90%	80%
65-74	91%	88%	88%
75 and over	85%	78%	82%

Note: Adapted from "Health & Socio-economic Inequalities," by R. Roberge, J. M. Berthelot, and M. Wolfson, 1995a, *Canadian Social Trends,* Summer, p. 18.

ries (Roberge, Berthelot, and Wolfson, 1995a). The Health Status Index was developed at McMaster University and combines descriptive and evaluative criteria to produce an overall health rating. The Health Status Index scores are highest among the lower age categories as would be expected, and they show a trend toward deterioration when viewed in terms of household income. This is particularly true for males in the 45 to 64 age ranges. Thus, this measure of both descriptive and subjective health indicators shows a significant relationship to income distribution as did the above longevity statistics.

A U.S. study conducted in Alameda County, California controlled for age, gender, race, smoking, alcohol consumption, sleep habits, physical activity, weight, blood pressure, and the presence of heart trouble, chest pain, diabetes, or cancer in comparing the risk of death among people with inadequate family incomes and with high family incomes. Results showed individuals with inadequate family incomes to be at a 2.1 times greater risk of death before adjustment for the control variables, and at a 1.6 times greater risk than their wealthier counterparts even after adjustment.

International comparisons also show a relationship between income levels and mortality rates. A study of the 11 member countries of the Organization for Economic Cooperation and Development showed not only support for the variance of rates of longevity by income, but also reported the impact of income distribution. This study concluded that the more equal the income distribution of a country, the higher the life expectancy. It reported that Norway, Sweden, and the Netherlands had the most equal income distributions and the highest life expectancies (National Council of Welfare, 1990).

The data presented in Table 5.4 show infant mortality rates in Canada for 1971 and 1986 by neighborhood income. As indicated, there is a decrease in infant mortality rates between 1971 and 1986 supporting, at least in part, the assumption that universal health coverage and improved health technology had a positive impact. However, these figures also show that the improvement in infant mortality overall did not affect significantly the risk of infant mortality relative to income levels. While all segments of the population showed a decreased risk of infant mortality, those risks remained highest in the lowest income levels.

The above summary of some overall health indicators for Canada provides support for a plausible interpretation that the universal health care system has had a beneficial impact on the overall health of Canadians. However, the summary demonstrates a negative relationship between income distribution and the health indicators. That is, it is apparent that issues of poverty and income distribution remain significant factors in health determination and begin to undermine the view of the universal, comprehensive health care system in Canada as a health panacea.

TABLE 5.4. Infant Deaths per 1,000 Births in Urban Canada by Neighborhood Income

	1971	1986
Poorest neighborhoods	20.0	10.5
Second poorest	16.6	8.0
Middle	15.2	7.7
Second richest	12.4	5.7
Richest neighborhoods	10.2	5.8
All neighborhoods	15.0	7.5

Note: Adapted from *Health, Health Care and Medicare*, p. 8, by The National Council of Welfare, Canada, 1990. Ottawa: Minister of Supply and Services.

The relationship between poverty and health has long been an area of interest for scholars and researchers. Antonovsky (1967) indicated an interest in the link between illness and poverty extending from the twelfth century. Other authors continue to indicate the higher likelihood of the poor to suffer both short-term and chronic illnesses (Badgley and Wolfe, 1992; Blackburn, 1991; Clarke, 1990; Graham, 1984; Mustard, 1994; Power, Manor, and Fox, 1991; Roberge, Berthelot, and Wolfson, 1995a). The material aspects of poverty such as poor nutrition, inadequate housing, lack of transportation, education level, lack of employment, and insufficient financial resources for medical services are all apparent contributors to this situation of poor health. Kane, Kasteler, and Gray (1976) indicated that health problems among the poor are traceable to the material situation of poverty, to the social structure of poverty, or to the aspects of the life outlook of poverty. There is, however, little or no research data to support the notion that the provision of universal, comprehensive health services significantly changes this situation.

Unfortunately, pre- and post-studies focusing upon implementation of a universal health care system in Canada are rare, and those which do exist are fraught with methodological problems including inconsistency in indicators of health and health service utilization. Badgley and Wolfe (1992) reported that well over 24 Canadian studies have been attempted in this area with results ranging from increased utilization of services by the poor, through to a decrease of services used by the poor, and an increase of services used by the more affluent. They go on to cite a pre-post Medicare implementation study conducted in Saskatchewan in the early 1960s which did show a lessening of the gap in service utilization between the rich and the poor, but also identified a tendency for the more affluent to utilize more sophisticated services and referrals to specialists. This tendency toward utilization of specialized services by wealthier individuals is supported by statistics showing higher utilization rates of specialized surgical procedures in the four provinces with the highest per capita income as compared to the four provinces with the lowest per capita income. The utilization rates were approximately double for the more affluent provinces in each category studied (Badgley and Wolfe, 1992).

Despite the methodological difficulties and inconclusiveness of studies in this area, the majority do provide indicators that the universal and comprehensive nature of the Canadian health care system does improve service utilization and early prevention. This is evident in the area of immunization and prenatal care. As noted in the United States-Canada comparison, deaths from infectious diseases and infant mortality rates are significantly less in Canada. These positive results were mirrored in a number of illness categories with death from cancer being the only anomaly. Even here, a recent meta-analysis concluded that when controlling for socioeconomic status, the comparisons for the two national populations showed that in low income areas, Canadian cases experienced advantaged survival rates at one- and five-year follow-ups, while no such between-country differentials were observed among their middle or high income groups (Gorey et al., 1997). Similarly, Gorey and Vena (1994) using a near-poverty SES measure found a clear association between SES and cancer incidence in the U.S. sample, while assumed racial differences were seen to be insignificant.

Many scholars and policymakers still express concern about differential usage of health services by the poor (Badgley and Wolfe, 1992; Davis, Gold, and Makuc, 1981; Doucette, Tholl, and Horne, 1994; Power, Manor, and Fox, 1991; Tallon and Block, 1988). They have pointed to cultural and/or attitudinal differences among the poor which contribute to this underutilization. These factors include differing definitions of health and illness, superstitions, lower priorities about health, fatalistic attitudes, and reduced self-esteem (Bergner and Yerby, 1976; Fries, 1995; Riessman, 1984). These and other sociocultural factors are seen to have a continuing impact even where universal health coverage exists. Higher rates of hospitalization, length of stay, and use of emergency facilities have been noted to be related to lower socioeconomic status. Similarly, lower rates of utilization of medical specialists, sophisticated treatments, and parahealth services such as dental, pharmacological, eye care, etc., have been associated directly with poverty (Badgley and Wolfe, 1992; Bergner and Yerby, 1976; Blackburn, 1991; Clarke, 1990; Davis, Gold, and Makuc, 1981; Dewar, 1994). While the existence of universally accessible health care narrows the gap in some areas of service utilization, the reality of poverty continues to have a significant negative effect on the health of Canada's population. The idea that universal health coverage provides a nation with a health panacea in reality is not supported by the data. It is probable that such a health care system is a necessary, but insufficient, approach to narrowing the health gap between rich and poor.

CURRENT TRENDS AND ISSUES

The mid-1990s find the Canadian health care system under ever increasing pressures from a variety of groups. For over a decade, political rhetoric and media attention have been focused upon national debt and deficit funding in an era of escalating costs (Madore, 1993). Contributing to these escalating costs are the issues of increased expectations for health services on the part of the Canadian population, coupled with the high cost of evolving sophisticated technologies (Beatty, 1993; Vayda and Deber, 1992). These pressures are further contributed to by the Canadian demographics of an increased proportion of aged persons combined with the decreasing birth rate, resulting in increasing demand and shrinking taxation resources. Not the least of these pressures is the state of the Canadian economy linked to and controlled by the emerging global economy and subject to repetitive recession and moves toward "downsizing" in the public and private sectors. Thus, we hear cries for cost containment happening simultaneously with expressed concerns about underfunding of the health care system.

In a political sense, these pressures seem to be giving rise to or influencing a number of other broad-based trends. There is a strong emergence of neoconservative ideology in the provincial and federal jurisdictions in Canada. Doyle (1995) points to an increasing view of health care as a major business and a tendency toward cartelization of health service delivery. Similarly, *The North American Free Trade Agreement* of 1991 placed pressure on the Canadian health care system to open opportunities for privatization and marketplace competition. To date, these pressures have translated into government efforts in the areas of cost containment and system streamlining.

As the political landscape changes, there is an ever increasing emphasis on personal responsibility. From a systems perspective, this has led to calls for reexamining the issues of extra billing by physicians, introduction of user fees, and development of a greater mix of private/public service delivery programs (a two-tiered system) (Evans, 1993; Vayda and Deber, 1992). While the rhetoric surrounding these issues overtly emphasizes the need for the affluent to contribute more to their own care, the underlying assumption is that of a return to a more residual social health and welfare ideology. The continued espousing of this residual view in other areas of social welfare programming may well spill over into issues surrounding universal, comprehensive health care of Canadians, and in turn, translate into an erosion of this system. Several authors have equated the Canadian populace's support for equity in health care accessibility to the Canadian identity (Beatty, 1993; Evans, 1993). However, these trends could render obsolete Federal Minister of Health Allan J. MacEachen's pronouncement that health care in Canada is a right, not a privilege (Badgley and Wolfe, 1992).

Studies, scholarly papers, and social policy reports have all identified the negative impacts of extra billing, user fees, and two-tiered systems upon the most disadvantaged in the society (Madore, 1993; Pollack, 1993; Vayda and Deber, 1992). The current impetus for system change has the most potential to undermine the health of poor Canadians and to reinforce the relationship between ill health and poverty. Even if the trend toward this type of change or the continued deterioration of service availability is resisted, there is a high potential that the health benefits of the system for the poor could be undermined by the deterioration in other social welfare programs.

There are a myriad of social welfare programs currently under review and/or revision within the context of cost reduction. Changes in social policy have already affected such institutional programs as old age security, unemployment insurance, worker's compensation, subsidized public housing and support for education programs. Within these programs, changes in eligibility, and availability and levels of support have the greatest impact upon the most disadvantaged in Canadian society. The current situation and trend toward deterioration in social welfare benefits to the poor can be best illustrated by reviewing social assistance financial benefits. Table 5.5 provides an overview of welfare benefits as percentages of provincial poverty lines and average incomes for 1994. Figures from New Brunswick, Ontario, and British Columbia were selected as being appropriate examples of the diverse regional differences in Canada, and Alberta figures are shown since significant efforts to reduce welfare costs in that province predate these figures.

When welfare benefits for 1994 are compared to 1986 using constant dollar adjustments, most Canadian provinces show only marginal improvements in benefit levels, with nine showing decreases in one or more of the categories of recipients. The province of Alberta which had undertaken welfare cost reductions showed decreases in all categories ranging from 40.3% for single employable individuals, to 16.1% for a couple with two children (National Council of Welfare, 1995). All jurisdictions in Canada are either currently implementing or planning to implement cost reduction measures. In April 1996, the province of Ontario instituted a 21.6% reduction in all categories of welfare benefits. The overall poverty rate in Canada for 1994 dropped slightly, but remained higher than the 1989 preresession rate. However, the depth of poverty estimate for the total Canadian population comparing 1980 to 1994 in 1994 dollars is up approximately 25%. In addition, the 1980 unemployment rate was 7.5% and the poverty rate for people 18 to 65 was 12.9%. In 1994, the unemployment rate was 10.4% and the poverty

TABLE 5.5. Welfare Incomes as Estimates of Poverty in Canada, 1994

	Total Welfare Income as % of Poverty Line	Welfare Income as % of Average Income
New Brunswick		
Single Employable	24%	15%
Single Parent, One Child	57%	53%
Couple, Two Children	46%	24%
Ontario		
Single Employable	55%	30%
Single Parent, One Child	80%	66%
Couple, Two Children	72%	34%
Alberta		
Single Employable	32%	21%
Single Parent, One Child	52%	42%
Couple, Two Children	56%	28%
British Columbia		
Single Employable	44%	25%
Single Parent, One Child	65%	52%
Couple, Two Children	57%	27%

Note: Adapted from *Welfare Incomes 1994,* pp. 30–36, by The National Council of Welfare, Canada, 1995. Ottawa: Minister of Supply and Services.

rate was 15.5% (National Council of Welfare, 1996). A pattern of increasing risk of poverty appears to be emerging that may not be reflected in welfare income statistics. While welfare recipients are not the only Canadians living in poverty or low socioeconomic conditions, their plight is illustrative of the circumstances for most. This trend toward a deterioration in the financial resources of the poor in Canada has significant implications for the health of this population as evidenced by the relationship between health and poverty already examined in this chapter.

IMPLICATIONS

The impact of overall decline in the Canadian economy, the participation in the emerging global economy, past debt with continuing deficits, and the shift to a more service-oriented economy all appear to be indicators of continued deterioration of resources for the less advantaged. There is a clear shrinkage in the middle class with many Canadians being displaced in a downward direction (McGilly, 1990). These factors make it dubious as to whether or not Canadian governments and the population as a whole will have sufficient commitment to sustain the universal, comprehensive health care system.

It has already been pointed out that in practice, when judged by utilization statistics and access to medical services not covered in the comprehensive health plan, a two-tiered health system already exists. It will be difficult to resist pressures toward privatization, user fees, and the formalization of two-tiered health systems for this country. Failure to do so will certainly have the most significant impact in terms of deteriorating health and lack of access to health care upon those with lower socioeconomic status. The current universal, comprehensive health care policies are incompatible with the reduction of overall economic resources and the need to cut deficits and debt.

It appears evident that the only avenue for sustaining a universal, comprehensive system within the context of reduction in expenditure is to explore reform of the system. It has been noted that an advantage of the single-payer system is its potential ability to control costs. If one discounts a move toward more privatization and self-payment, then we are left with a need to exert more control over service providers and service utilization. It is feasible that managed health care initiatives in the United States (such as HMOs and PPOs) could be initiated within the system. Since the Canadian system is a public program, this would move it closer to the reality of socialized medicine. In 1996, the Ontario government initiated physician billing caps and reductions to physician malpractice insurance premiums, and began discussion of limiting patient choice in physician selection. Most governments, including Canada's, have watched intently the research and scholarship in the state of Oregon dealing with health care prioritization (Wong, 1994). It now seems plausible that the past views from outside Canada, erroneously indicating lack of choice in physician and facility, government determination of appropriate treatment, and health service rationing or prioritization of availability, may be future realities. Experience has taught us that bureaucratic or government regulated processes limiting access and eligibility have usually most disadvantaged the poor (Morton and Loos, 1995). This situation, along with the previously noted cultural tendencies of the poor toward reduced utilization of health services, would combine to take the biggest toll on the health of the least advantaged in our society.

This possible system reform or the continued decline of comprehensive health services in Canada is even more apparent when one examines the circumstances of cohorts within this disadvantaged population. The 1980s and 1990s have seen continued growth in the numbers of children living in poverty, an increased number of elderly persons without an improvement of the proportion living below the poverty line, and little or no improvement to the economic resources of the disabled. The residual view currently being expressed through neoconservative ideology and shifts in public policy assumes that individuals in the lower socioeconomic strata could be encouraged to look after themselves if reduced public support occurred. However, this view ignores the reality that this segment of the population contains a high proportion of children, elderly, and disabled persons who do not fit this ideological view.

In order to plan, monitor, and, potentially, avoid a deterioration in the overall health of Canadians at all socioeconomic levels, it will be necessary to have sound information based on empirical data. A report by the National Council of Welfare (1990) recommended research be undertaken focusing upon enhancing the understanding of the health gap between rich and poor through regular health status surveys of Canadians. In addition, it is recommended that further study be initiated exploring the causal factors for the health gap and, most important, for developing strategies for reducing the gap (Levine, 1994). Given the circumstances facing both federal and provincial governments in the mid-1990s, these recommendations appear even more salient.

REFERENCES

Adler, N.E., Boyce, T., Chesney, M.A., and Cohen, S. (1994). Socioeconomic status and health: The challenge of the gradient. *American-Psychologist, 49*, 25–24.

Anderson, N.B., and Armstead, C.A. (1995). Toward understanding the association of socioeconomic status and health: A new challenge for the biopsychosocial approach, *Psychosomatic Medicine, 57*(3), 213–225.

Antonovsky, A. (1967). Social class, life expectancy and overall mortality. *Millbank Memorial Fund Quarterly, 45*, 31–73.

Badgley, R.F., and Wolfe, S. (1992). Equity and health care. In C.D. Naylor (ed.), *Canadian health care and the state* (pp. 193–237). Montreal, Canada: McGill-Queen's University Press.

Beatty, P. (1993). A comparison of our two systems. In A. Bennett and O. Adams (eds.), *Looking north of health: What we can learn from Canada's health care system* (pp. 28–39). San Francisco, CA: Jossey-Bass.

Bellamy, D., and Irving, A. (1995). Pioneers. In J.C. Turner and F.J. Turner (eds.), *Canadian social welfare* (third ed.) (pp. 89–117). Scarborough, Ontario: Allyn & Bacon Canada.

Bergner, L., and Yerby, A.S. (1976). Low income and barriers to use of health services. In R.L. Kane, J.M. Kasteler, and R.M. Gray (eds.) *The health gap: Medical services and the poor* (pp. 27–39). New York: Springer Publishing Company.

Blackburn, C. (1991). *Poverty and health: Working with families*. Milton Keynes: Open University Press.

Clarke, J.N. (1990). *Health, illness, and medicine in Canada*. Toronto, Ontario: McClelland & Stewart.

Davis, K., Gold, M., and Makuc, D. (1981). Access to health care for the poor: Does the gap remain? *Annual Review of Public Health, 2*, 159–182.

Dewar, D. (1994). Variations in health service demand under alternative reimbursement systems. In J.A. Boan (ed.), *Proceedings of the fifth Canadian conference on health economics* (pp. 184–205). Regina, Saskatchewan: Canadian Plains Research Center, University of Regina.

Doucette, K., Tholl, W., and Horne, J. (1994). Consumers as "agents of reform" in Canadian health care delivery. In J.A. Boan (ed.), *Proceedings of the fifth Canadian conference on health economics* (pp. 138–159). Regina, Saskatchewan: Canadian Plains Research Center, University of Regina.

Doyle, R. (1995, July). *The Re-emergence of cartelisation in the social welfare services*. Paper presented at the Conference on International Social Welfare at the University of Calgary, Canada.

Evans, R.G. (1993). Health care in the Canadian community. In A. Bennett and O. Adams (eds.), *Looking north of health: What we can learn from Canada's health care system* (pp. 1–27). San Francisco, CA: Jossey-Bass.

Fries, J.F. (1995). The cost corollary: Reducing need and demand for medical services. Special section: Are mind-body variables a central factor linking socioeconomic status and health? *Advances, 11*, 9–12.

Gorey, K.M., Holowaty, E.J, Fehringer, G., Laukkanen, E., Moskowitz, A., Webster, D.J., and Richter, N. (1997). An international comparison of cancer survival: Toronto, Ontario and Detroit, Michigan metropolitan areas, *American Journal of Public Health*, July.

Gorey, K.M., and Vena, J.E. (1994). The association of near poverty status with cancer incidence among black and white adults. *Journal of Community Health*, *20*, 359–366.

Graham, H. (1984). *Women, health and the family*. Brighton: Wheatsheaf Books.

Kane, R.L., Kasteler, J.M., and Gray, R.M. (eds.) (1976). *The health gap: Medical services and the poor*. New York: Springer Publishing Company.

Kunitz, S.J. (1992). Socialism and social insurance in the United States and Canada. In C.D. Naylor (ed.), *Canadian health care and the state* (pp. 104–124). Montreal, Canada: McGill-Queen's University Press.

Lepore, G. (1994). *Your money or your life*. Kingston, Ontario: Kashtan Press.

Levine, S. (1994). If our government really cared about health. *Social Policy*, *24*, 6–12.

Madore, O. (1993). *Health care financing: User participation*. Ottawa: Canada Communication Group.

McGilly, F.J. (1990). *An introduction to Canada's public social services: Understanding income and health programs*. Toronto, Ontario: McClelland & Stewart.

Morton, A.M., and Loos, C. (1995). Does universal health care coverage mean universal accessibility? Examining the Canadian experience of poor, prenatal women. *Women's Health Issues*, *5*, 139–142.

Mustard, F. (1994). Economic growth, prosperity and the determinants of health. In J.A. Boan (ed.), *Proceedings of the fifth Canadian conference on health economics* (pp. 39–46). Regina, Saskatchewan: Canadian Plains Research Center, University of Regina.

Nair, C., Karim, R., and Nyers, C. (1992). Health care and health status: A Canadian–United States statistical comparison. *Health Reports*, *4*(2), 175–182.

National Council of Welfare (1990). *Health, health care and Medicare*. Ottawa: Minister of Supply and Services Canada 1990.

National Council of Welfare (1995). *Welfare incomes 1994*. Ottawa: Minister of Supply and Services Canada 1995.

National Council of Welfare (1996). *Poverty profile 1994*. Ottawa: Minister of Supply and Services Canada 1996.

Pollack, R. (1993). Eleven lessons from Canada's health care system. In A. Bennett and O. Adams (eds.), *Looking north of health: What we can learn from Canada's health care system* (pp. 142–176). San Francisco, CA: Jossey-Bass.

Power, C., Manor, O., and Fox, J. (1991). *Health and class: The early years*. London: Chapman & Hall.

Riessman, C.K. (1984). The use of health services by the poor: Are there any promising models? *Social Policy*, *14*, 30–40.

Roberge, R., Berthelot, J.M., and Wolfson, M. (1995a). Health & socio-economic inequalities. *Canadian Social Trends, Summer*, 15–19.

Roberge, R., Berthelot, J.M., and Wolfson, M. (1995b). The health utility index: Measuring health differences in Ontario by socioeconomic status. *Health Reports*, *7*(2), 25–43.

Schiller, B.R. (1989). *The economics of poverty & discrimination* (Fifth ed.). Englewood Cliffs, NJ: Prentice Hall.

Summer, L. (1994). The escalating number of uninsured in the United States. *International Journal of Health Services*, *24*, 409–413.

Tallon, J.R., and Block, R. (1988). Changing patterns of health insurance coverage: Special concerns for women. In C.A. Perales and L.S. Young (eds.), *Women, health, and poverty* (pp. 119–138). Binghamton, NY: The Haworth Press.

Terris, M. (1990). Lessons from Canada's health program. *Technology Review*, *93*, 19–34.

Turner, J. (1995). The historical base. In J.C. Turner and F.J. Turner (eds.), *Canadian social welfare* (3rd ed.) (pp. 75–88). Scarborough, Ontario: Allyn & Bacon Canada.

Vayda, E., and Deber, R. (1992). The Canadian health-care system: A developmental overview. In C.D. Naylor (ed.), *Canadian health care and the state* (pp. 125–140). Montreal, Canada: McGill-Queen's University Press.

Wilkins, K. (1995). Causes of death: How the sexes differ. *Health Reports*, *7*, 33–43.

Wong, A.M.F. (1994). The Oregon approach to health care: Its applicability to Canada. In J.A. Boan (ed.), *Proceedings of the fifth Canadian conference on health economics* (pp. 47–58). Regina, Saskatchewan: Canadian Plains Research Center, University of Regina.

Zambrana, R.E. (1988). A research agenda on issues affecting poor and minority women: A model for understanding their health needs. In C.A. Perales and L.S. Young (eds.), *Women, health, and poverty* (pp. 137–160). Binghamton, NY: The Haworth Press.

PART II:
IMPACTS, INFLUENCES, RESULTS,
AND CONSEQUENCES

Health care policies and services purport to produce a set of outcomes in which the health needs of poor people are being met. In Section II, these efforts call attention to the unique circumstances of poor people, and to being sensitive to racial, ethnic, cultural, gender, and disability factors, as well as other unique or vulnerable populations. The authors in this section demonstrate the continuing efforts and dedication of many individuals, programs, and services to intervene on behalf of the poor, and to work toward their inclusion in the health care agenda of the United States. However, as a whole these chapters illustrate clearly the root of this problem, which has to do with making incremental and idiosyncratic modifications but not significantly changing the fundamental structure of the medical and health care system as it relates to serving the needs of poor people.

Chapter 6

Who Bears the Burden
of Uncompensated Hospital Care?

Howard P. Tuckman
Cyril F. Chang

INTRODUCTION

The medical treatment of persons who cannot pay is normally referred to as "charity care," "uncompensated care," "no-charge care," or "indigent care." Irrespective of how such care is labelled, it has been a source of controversies in both the news media and public policy debates. Recently, a great deal has been written about the magnitude and consequences of the indigent care "problem" and about how to finance such care (Aday, Anderson, and Fleming, 1980; Brown, 1983; Eastaugh, 1987; Feder, Hadley, and Mullner, 1984a, 1984b; Kelly, 1985). To date, relatively little attention has been paid to the issues surrounding how to assess the fairness of the existing distribution of the financial burden. This chapter both identifies the various sources of funds that are available for financing indigent care and explores the major issues which arise in evaluating the fairness issues of indigent patient care.

THE QUESTION OF INDIGENT CARE BURDEN

To investigate the distribution of the indigent care burden and to assess its fairness, a necessary first step is to identify the various

This chapter was originally published in *Journal of Health and Social Policy,* Vol. 2(1) 1990.

The authors wish to acknowledge the support of the Avron B. and Robert F. Fogelman Academic Excellence Fund, which partially funded this study.

parties that bear the financial burden of such care. Although indigent patients receive their medical care in a hospital, the provider may or may not eventually bear the financial burden. If a hospital pays for indigent services out of its own reserves or endowment funds, that hospital bears the burden. However, hospitals are limited in the amount that they can pay out of their own funds. Hence, they will seek other sources to share the burden with. If another source is found, at least a portion of the burden is shifted to that party. In this case, the burden shifts from the hospital to a third party.

A hospital's ability to find funds to pay for indigent care rests upon its ingenuity and its access to financial resources (Herzlinger and Krasker, 1987). We have identified the following sources of funds for financing indigent care: improvements in operating efficiency, cross-subsidization and price discrimination, reduced hospital expenditures, subsidies from endowments, subsidies from unrelated businesses, outside donations, direct public payments, and implicit public subsidies. As the discussion below will suggest, the approaches that hospitals take to sharing the financial burden of indigent care play a significant role in determining who bears the ultimate burden of this care.

WHO BEARS THE BURDEN?

Improved Efficiency

Under certain circumstances, an increase in patient volume resulting from the admission of indigent patients can improve efficiencies which lower the cost of operation. For example, if increased volume makes it possible to use operating rooms and the other costly facilities more effectively, average operating cost will fall. Chang and Tuckman (1986) documented such savings for Tennessee hospitals.

When greater operating efficiency is achieved, it may be possible for hospitals to use the reduced average costs of operation to create a pool of funds that can be used for quality improvements, indigent care, or future capital expansion. In this instance, use of funds for indigent care creates a burden in the form of opportunities foregone by not using the savings for other purposes. Those who might have benefited from the alternative use of the funds then bear the burden imposed by the treatment of indigents. Alternatively, if average cost reductions are reflected in lower prices to patients (an option which is feasible but not likely), current patients and their insurers may bear the burden in the form of lower prices foregone because hospitals have used the savings to treat indigents.

Cross-Subsidization and Price Discrimination

It has been alleged that hospitals engage in cross-subsidization by overcharging patients with an ability-to-pay (usually those with adequate insurance coverage) to cover the costs of providing care to indigents (Clark, 1980; Ginsburg and Sloan, 1984). Because the costs of treating one group of patients are shifted to another, the practice of cross-subsidization is also referred to as "cost shifting" in the health services research literature. Cross-subsidization may also take place if hospitals use profits from business activities only tangential to health care (e.g., the hospital gift shop or laundry) to subsidize money-losing services and procedures. Evidence on the existence and prevalence of the several forms of cross-subsidization is mixed because the data necessary to measure this practice are scarce (Bazzoli, 1986; Ginsburg and Sloan, 1984; Hadley and Feder, 1985; Sloan and Becker, 1984).

Hospitals may also engage in price discrimination to cover the costs of indigent care, raising the price of highly price-inelastic services and procedures while leaving the price of price-sensitive services and procedures unchanged. The resulting surpluses from the higher prices charged may be used to finance indigent care. Although data are insufficient to permit a conclusive answer to the question of how much price discrimination takes place, it seems likely that those with severe illnesses, which require intensive and specialized care, and their insurers bear at least a portion of the costs of the indigent care provided by the hospital.

Reduced Expenditure

At least some evidence supports the view that hospitals pass the cost of indigent care to their employees. This is not surprising given that labor costs represent a significant part of most hospital operating budgets. Hadley and Feder (1985) present evidence that those hospitals with a need to shift costs also reduce the number of their personnel and postpone pay increases. The former lowers the costs of the delivery of services and it may also lower the quality of the services offered. The latter lowers short-run costs and it may raise turnover and employee costs in the long run. Moreover, Hadley and Feder (1985) find that financially distressed hospitals tend to reduce the amount of indigent care they provide, passing the burden of indigent care onto other hospitals and/or back to indigents. This practice suggests that the distribution of indigent care may grow more concentrated if hospitals experience financial exigency. Hospitals may also choose to postpone expenditures for new capital equipment or physical plants. Over time, this passes the burden to future patients in the form of lower quality facilities and inferior equipment, to physicians in the form of fewer accessible beds and less amenities from the hospital, and to indigents in the form of fewer opportunities for adequate care (Feder, Hadley, and Mullner, 1984b).

Subsidies from Endowment Funds

As discussed above, a number of hospitals, especially not-for-profits (NOPROs), maintain some type of reserve and/or endowment funds. Funds of this type are used to accumulate capital for expansion, to provide a cushion against temporary downturns in revenue, to ensure the perpetuation of the institution, to fund charitable care, and to store funds against future operating needs (Chang and Tuckman, 1988a). Hansmann (1986) and Chang and Tuckman (1988b) have argued that these funds are more likely to be found at NOPRO hospitals than at for-profit (FOPRO) or government (GOV) hospitals. They also have pointed out that these funds can potentially be an important source of charitable funds, as is the case with many research-oriented hospitals. To the extent that indigent care is financed from endowment funds, the burden is borne by the initial donors of the funds, and in the form of opportunities foregone by using the funds to finance indigent care rather than to engage in research, improve facilities, offer staff perquisites, subsidize unprofitable services or procedures, or upgrade staff and equipment. Some researchers have argued that NOPROs use at least a portion of their net profits to raise salaries and positions (Clark, 1980). To the extent that this is the case, increases in indigent care financed out of internal funds will be partially borne by the hospital staff in the form of compensation and advancement opportunities foregone.

To the extent that hospitals use their reserves to finance indigent care in lieu of capital expansion, the burden may fall on future users of the facilities. The problem is particularly acute for NOPROs because they have difficulty raising funds in equity markets (Institute of Medicine, 1986). In contrast, GOVs tend to rely on public funding to finance their expansions while FOPROs raise funds in equity markets. If FOPROs choose to offer indigent care, they must be careful. A large indigent effort can impact on FOPRO capital expansion through its effect on the financial ratios that lenders use to judge the risk involved in investing capital in a venture. Should these ratios deteriorate as a result of substantial indigent care burden, a FOPRO hospital could find itself shut out of the equity market. Should this happen, this would impact not only on future users of that hospital but also on the hospital's stockholders. The above discussion suggests that viewed from a capital expansion point of view, state and local government hospitals (GOVs) are probably in the best positions to make a large indigent care efforts because they rely mainly on government appropriations for their capital needs. However, the large federal budget deficits and the pressures on state and local government funds will continue to limit the abilities of GOV hospitals to finance indigent care.

Subsidies from Unrelated Businesses

In recent years, many hospitals have expanded their operations to include such businesses as wellness and fitness centers, home health agencies, nursing homes, and even business activities unrelated to health care such as maternity clothing, data processing, and real estate. While some FOPRO hospitals have diversified in this manner, NOPROs are the entities most likely to have reorganized in ways that permit subsidies from the surpluses of affiliated NOPRO and FOPRO subsidiaries. These subsidies may then be used to diversify a hospital's financial base, to supplement its reserves, and/or to allow entry into new markets. To the extent that subsidies are provided out of profits of these businesses, the burden is in the form of opportunities foregone by spending these funds on indigents rather than on other health or nonhealth ventures. As the corporate structures of hospitals grow more complex, it has become increasingly difficult to identify the types of opportunities given up when funds are diverted to indigent care. It has also become more difficult to identify the actual dollars transferred among entities.

Donations

Because of their tax-exempt status, NOPROs are eligible to receive tax-deductible donations. While FOPROs can also receive donations, these contributions are not tax deductible and donations to GOVs, while not unheard of, are rare. Irrespective of ownership type, donations are an insignificant source of revenue, amounting to less than 1% of the revenues of hospitals in 1986 (American Hospital Association, 1986). Since 1969, the Internal Revenue Service has not required that the provision of indigent care be an explicit prerequisite for tax-exempt status (Bromberg, 1970). Hence, NOPRO donations need not be used for indigent care but may instead serve to expand capital facilities, improve the quality of service delivery, augment salaries or number of staff, and/or raise the level of the hospital's endowment fund(s).

Advocates of a greater role for NOPROs as financiers of health care argue that it is a contradiction for paying patients to pay for care that they do not receive in a charitable hospital, that NOPROs exist in part to relieve the government of the burden of health care, that free or below-cost care should be a necessary part of a NOPRO's mission, and/or that NOPROs should be more charitable than FOPROs (Bromberg, 1970; Herzlinger and Krasker, 1987; and Taylor and O'Donnell, 1988). To the extent that indigent care is financed through tax-deductible donations, the burden of indigent care is borne both by donors and taxpayers. The relative burden assumed by each is determined by the provisions governing deductibility under federal and state income tax laws.

Direct Public Payments

Public payments to finance the provision of health care are made to individuals and to hospitals. In the latter case, government indigent care programs serve both to create an incentive for hospitals to treat indigents (e.g., Medicare/Medicaid) and to target particular groups for treatment (e.g., funds for adolescent services) (Bazzoli, 1986). These payments are often accompanied by one or more constraints on the way that hospitals can use funds and/or on the size of the reimbursement that they can receive. When public funds are distributed for indigent care, the burden is passed onto taxpayers and is distributed according to the existing mix of taxes and their incidence (the distributional effects of taxation). However, the burden is more complex if these funds do not cover the full cost of the care dispensed to recipients. That portion of care which is not covered by public payments must be financed by the hospital from the other sources enumerated above. Depending on which sources of finance are chosen, the uncompensated portion of the care can be shifted back to labor or capital, financed through increased efficiency, or passed forward to current or future patients.

Implicit Public Subsidies

A number of authors have argued that NOPRO hospitals receive implicit public subsidies which should be used to finance a higher level of indigent care than they actually provide (Clark, 1980; Herzlinger and Krasker, 1987). Such subsidies include, among other things, exemption from federal corporate income tax, state and local sales and property taxes, free or minimal cost for the use of public land, lower cost mailing privileges, and access to volunteer labor. Public subsidies to not-for-profit organizations have a long history in the United States (Hansmann, 1986). However, the rationale for these subsidies has been periodically challenged (Clark, 1980; Herzlinger and Krasker, 1987; Taylor and O'Donnell, 1988). A central issue is whether the provision of health care is in itself of sufficient benefit to the community to justify the special treatment that NOPROs receive or whether a substantial level of charitable care should also be a prerequisite if a hospital is to receive implicit public subsidies (Bromberg, 1970). If the former answer is valid, NOPROs need not demonstrate a large amount of indigent care to justify their nonprofit status. If the latter answer is chosen, a need exists to answer the question, "How much charity care is enough?"

It should also be noted that public funding can indirectly stimulate the provision of indigent care. For example, the Hospital Survey and Construction Act (Hill-Burton) of 1946 offered federal funds for construction and modernization of hospitals on the condition that the hospitals receiving these funds agreed to provide a certain amount of indigent care each year. Bazzoli (1986) notes that in 1984, approximately 3,000 hospitals delivered $3 billion in charity care in fulfillment of Hill-Burton obligations.

The effect of these types of public subsidies is to reduce the cost of operation for recipient hospitals relative to what it would be in their absence. The cost savings from these subsidies are potentially available to provide "charitable" care but there is evidence that the additional care provided by NOPRO hospitals is at best limited (Clark, 1980). The burden of providing these subsidies is borne primarily by the taxpayers and is estimated to be in the billions (Herzlinger and Krasker, 1987). However, an accurate estimation of the impact of these subsidies involves resolution of the issue addressed above; namely, whether such subsidies result in a pool of funds which lie dormant in endowment funds or whether they give rise to increases in operating costs which either raise quality or are dissipated by the inefficient use of capital.

In Sum

The above discussion of who bears the burden of hospital-provided indigent care suggests at least three insights. First, no simple answer exists to this question. Much depends on how hospitals choose to react to a rise in their indigent load, on the competitive conditions they face, and on the sources of funds available to them to cover indigent care costs. Second, while legislatures and regulatory bodies can mandate that hospitals provide a certain amount of indigent care, they cannot ensure that hospitals will be the ultimate financiers of this care nor can they currently identify the actual bearers of the burden. Third, given differences in hospital policies regarding the use of donations, willingness to cross-subsidize and price discriminate, cost cutting, fund raising, use of unrelated business funds, and willingness to accept public largesses, it is likely that major differences will continue to exist in the ability of individual hospitals to assume the burden of providing indigent care.

TOWARD A FAIRER JUDGMENT
OF THE DISTRIBUTION OF INDIGENT BURDEN

The analysis presented above raises several caveats concerning our ability to accurately judge the fairness of the current apportionment of indigent care among hospitals. First, different impressions of the fairness of indigent care effort can be drawn because fairness depends on how indigent care is defined and measured on the one hand, and on the prevailing societal view on how the total indigent care effort ought to be distributed on the other hand. Without a consensus on how effort should be judged, fairness, like beauty, will remain in the eye of the beholder.

It is far easier to identify who provides indigent care than it is to identify who bears the burden of this care. It is also unlikely that the problems inherent in measuring who bears the burden of indigent care will be resolved in the near future. When hospitals are asked to finance indigent care out of "own" revenues, they will use every means at their disposal to cover the costs of this care in ways that meet their individual needs. The needs of hospitals differ, as do the sources of funds available to them. This hampers the ability of decision makers to judge the fairness of the final outcome.

Differences in the degree of competition in markets, in third-party reimbursement policies in different states and geographic areas, in attitudes of governing boards and regulatory agencies, and in financial position of providers all serve to shape the strategies that hospitals use to finance indigent care. This is particularly true for urban hospitals (Feder, Hadley, and Mullner, 1984a). As conditions change, so do the sources of finance and the incidence of indigent care burden. These all add to the difficulty of assigning specific numbers in answer to the question, "Who bears the final burden of indigent care?"

At a minimum, policy makers should recognize that simply because a hospital provides a given dollar amount of indigent care, it is not necessarily true that the same level of financial burden is borne by the hospital. Because hospitals are highly adaptable, and because costs can be passed on, the final resting place of indigent care burden differs from where it originates. While it is easy to argue that hospitals are inefficient and that the belt tightening brought about by the need to finance indigent care will ultimately benefit society, limits exist on hospitals' abilities to provide charitable care. As some hospitals assume a larger burden in financing indigent care, it is increasingly likely that persons associated with these hospitals will assume a greater part of the burden of providing that care.

As competition increases among health care providers, many hospitals will find it difficult (and/or will be unwilling) to fund indigent care from the sources enumerated above. Ultimately, more hospitals will transfer indigents to a few hospitals and this will centralize the provision of such care even more than it is currently. Should this occur, the ultimate providers of indigent care in our society are likely to be the large urban government hospitals affiliated with medical schools. It may be that this is the fairest and most efficient solution from society's point of view but consensus is lacking on this point at the present time. It would be a pity if such a development emerged without explicit consideration of the alternatives, and it would be both unfortunate and unfair if these public hospitals were left with insufficient funds to meet the demands placed upon them.

REFERENCES

Aday, L., Anderson, R., and Fleming, G. (1980). *Health Care in the United States: Equitable for Whom?* Beverly Hills, CA: Sage Publications.

American Hospital Association. (1986). *Hospital Statistics, 1986 Edition.* Chicago, IL: American Hospital Association.

Bazzoli, G.J. (1986). Health Care for the Indigent: Overview of Critical Issues. *Health Service Research, 21*(3), 354–393.

Bromberg, R.S. (1970). The Charitable Hospital. *Catholic University Law Review, 20*(2), 237–258.

Brown, E. (1983). Public Hospitals on the Brink: Their Problems and Their Options. *Journal of Health Politics, Policy, and Law, 7*(4), 927–944.

Chang, C.F., and Tuckman, H.P. (1986). Structure of Production, Output Level, and the Cost of Hospital Care: Are For-Profit Hospitals More Effective? *American Statistical Association Proceedings of the Business and Economic Statistics Section.*

_____. (1988a). The Profits of Not-For-Profit Hospitals. *Journal of Health Politics, Policy, and Law, 13*(3), 547–564.

_____. (1988b). On The Role and Use of Endowment Funds. Unpublished manuscript, Memphis State University.

Clark, R. (1980). Does The Nonprofit Form Fit the Hospital Industry? *Harvard Law Review,* 93, 1417–1489.

Eastaugh, S.R. (1987). *Financing Health Care.* Dover, MA: Auburn Publishing House.

Feder, J., Hadley, J., and Mullner, R. (1984a). Poor People and Poor Hospitals: Implications for Public Policy. *Journal of Health Politics, Policy and Law,* 9(2), 237–250.

_____. (1984b). Falling Through the Cracks: Poverty, Insurance Coverage, and Hospitals' Care to the Poor, 1980–82. *Milbank Memorial Fund Quarterly,* 62(4), 544–566.

Ginsburg, P., and Sloan, F. (1984). Hospital Cost Shifting. *The New England Journal of Medicine, 310*(14), 893–898.

Hadley, J., and Feder, J. (1985). Hospital Cost Shifting and Care for the Uninsured. *Health Affairs, 4*(3), 67–80.

Hansmann, H. (1986). The Role of Nonprofit Enterprise. In *The Economics of Nonprofit Institutions,* edited by S. Rose-Ackerman. New York: Oxford University Press, 367–393.

Herzlinger, R., and Krasker, W. (1987). Who Profits from Nonprofits? *Harvard Business Review,* 13, 93–105.

Institute of Medicine (1986). Financial Capital and Health Care Growth Trends. In *For-Profit Enterprise in Health Care.* Washington, DC: National Academy Press.

Kelly, J. (1985). Provision of Charity Care by Urban Voluntary Hospitals. In *Hospitals and the Uninsured Poor: Measuring and Paying for Uncompensated Care,* edited by S. Rogers, A. Rouseau, and S. Nesbitt. New York: United Hospital Fund, pp. 49–69.

Sloan, F., and Becker, E. (1984). Cross-Subsidies and Payment for Hospital Care. *Journal of Health Politics, Policy and Law,* 8(4), 660–685.

Taylor, J., and O'Donnell, J. (1988). Property Taxation of a Not-For-Profit Hospital: A Case Study. *Hospital and Health Services Administration, 33*(1), 111–119.

Chapter 7

Medical Indigency and Inner-City Hospital Care: Patient Dumping, Emergency Care, and Public Policy

Mitchell F. Rice

INTRODUCTION

Changes in financing of the American health care system during the last few years have resulted in major gaps in the "safety net" which protects the poor/indigent from the ravages of disease and illness. These changes have favored a shift toward market competitiveness as a means of controlling rising health care costs. As this approach has become more characteristic of the American health care system, the problems of the medically indigent have become more pronounced. The severity of medical indigency has led some 30 states to establish task forces to study the problem (Perkins et al., 1986). Nowhere is the problem more acute than in the growing lack of private for-profit hospital care for the medically indigent. About two-thirds of the hospitals in the country are private institutions.

Public and/or charity hospital use has been on an increase in recent years. This increase can be attributed to several factors: (1) changes in Medicaid eligibility requirements; (2) changes in Medicare reimburse-

This chapter was originally published in *Journal of Health & Social Policy*, Vol. 1(2) 1989.

The author wishes to acknowledge research assistance provided by graduate student Carl Primeaux.

ment schedules; (3) a general increase in the number of uninsured individuals; and (4) the alarming increase in the transfer of uninsured and underinsured patients from private for-profit hospitals to public/charity hospitals, a phenomenon known as "dumping." Other terminologies used to describe this phenomenon are "case shifting" and "economically motivated transfers" (Duncan and Vogel, 1988).

Hospital dumping has generated considerable attention in both the health and political arenas. The attention has magnified because of the increasing number of transfer patients requiring emergency care upon arrival at a public hospital. In some cases private for-profit hospitals have delayed treatment or flatly refused to treat uninsured or underinsured individuals and, as a result, death or permanent disability has occurred (see *The Wall Street Journal,* 1985; Schiff et al., 1985; Klaidman, 1986; Wrenn, 1985; Friedman, 1982; *Chicago Tribune,* 1982; *Des Moines Register,* 1982). Yet, for years the transfer of patients from one hospital to another had been considered appropriate (and still is) when patients need special care and/or services that are unavailable at the referring hospital.

On February 5, 1985 and February 6, 1985, *CBS Evening News* and *ABC Evening News,* respectively, reported the following incident. A 34-year-old uninsured black man with a wound from a knife that penetrated his skull was denied emergency neurosurgery at a private hospital. Though the hospital began treatment in the emergency room and had complete neurosurgical facilities, the patient was refused further care. Following transfer to another facility (two other hospitals refused to accept him), the patient died.

In other cases, private for-profit hospitals have provided only a modicum of care to stabilize the patient for transfer to a public hospital where upon arrival the patient's health has deteriorated to such a point that death or permanent disability occurs. In Chicago, for example, nearly 25% of the transfers to Cook County Hospital were in unstable condition and their death rate was two-and-one-half times higher than that of other patients. Further, in areas where indigency or public aid is not accepted as a reason for transfer, a transferring hospital may often misrepresent the reason for transfer. That is, a hospital may claim the transfer is purely for a medical reason.

Why do private for-profit hospitals transfer (dump) uninsured and underinsured patients to public hospitals? Do private for-profit hospitals have legal and moral obligations to provide emergency care to all who seek their services? This chapter addresses these questions. These questions are especially noteworthy since the profit margin of the private hospital sector (at least in 1984) in the United States is at its highest in 20 years (Ansell and Schiff, 1987).[1] The chapter also discusses governmental policy responses to the dumping issue.

THE DUMPING PHENOMENON

Ansell and Schiff (1987:1500) define "patient dumping as the denial of or limitation in the provision of medical services to a patient for economic reasons and the referral of that patient elsewhere." Dumped patients can be divided into two categories: inpatient and outpatient.

> Inpatient dumping involves ambulatory hospital to hospital transfer of patients too sick to be discharged but stable enough to transfer. Outpatient dumping involves those patients who require hospitalization but who may safely be discharged. (*Americans at Risk,* 1985:30–36, testimony by Dr. G. Schiff)

Outpatient dumping is difficult to quantify and study because there is little or no follow-up of such patients. It is difficult to ascertain if an individual has been refused treatment as an outpatient at an emergency care facility.

While dumping can occur in any part of a hospital, it most commonly occurs in the emergency room. This is not surprising since emergency room use has risen rapidly in recent years. By 1984 some 160 million visits were expected to the emergency room, an increase of 151 million visits or 1,800% since 1954 (Wing and Campbell, 1985). While up to 30% of a hospital's admissions may come from the emergency room (Wing and Campbell, 1985), by dumping unwanted patients a hospital may exercise judgement regarding who it will or will not treat. Dumping can result from both hospital policies and practices. Examples of hospital policies and practices may include requiring advance payment, refusing patients who do not have a physician on the hospital's staff, refusing to accept Medicaid patients, and long delays in treatment. For minorities, especially blacks, dumping has serious implications in health care. For large numbers of blacks, the hospital emergency room is the provider of last resort (Seger, 1983). Rice (1985/86:66) notes that:

> More often than not the . . . hospital's emergency department serves as the entry point into the health-care system for inner-city blacks and the poor. The emergency department acts as the primary care center, preventive care center, trauma center, and intensive care center all at once for the indigent patient such as the feverish baby, the shooting victim, the high-risk pregnant mother, the premature neonate, the unwedded teenage mother, and so on.

A study of 26 urban public hospitals in 12 states and the District of Columbia involving 1,066 patients indicated that dumping had become a widespread phenomenon. The study pointed out that at least 15% of emergency transfer patients to public hospitals qualified as dumping. Some hospital analysts suggested that this figure may have been considerably higher. For example, in Washington, DC, transfers from private hospitals to DC General Hospital increased from 169 to about 1,000 annually between the years 1981 and 1984 (Greensberg, 1984). The number of transfers to Cook County Hospital in Chicago increased by more than five times between 1980 and 1983, from 1,295 to 6,769 (Schiff et al., 1986; Dowell, 1984).

In Texas, dumping has been recently documented at more than 40 hospitals. While hospital dumping has been more pronounced in urban areas, it has been reportedly occurring in smaller cities and rural areas (Ansberry, 1988). Further, the rights of indigent patients are ignored when a private hospital makes a decision to transfer. At Cook County hospital only 6% of transferred patients provided written consent for transfer (Schiff et al., 1986).

In some states such as Texas, Florida, Tennessee, and Kentucky where profit-oriented hospital chains have proliferated and acquired a large share of the market, dumping has been an extremely serious problem (Relman, 1986). In Texas, private hospitals compromise about one-third of the total hospitals in the state (Berg, 1983). Even a Medicaid recipient is not immune from dumping. A study of 467 patient transfers to Cook County Hospital found that 46% were recipients of public aid (Schiff et al., 1986). Another 46% had no insurance. Further, the study suggests that insurance status may be closely associated with race. Schiff et al. (1986) found that 89% of the transfers involve minority members (blacks and Hispanics). The study also estimated the cost of care provided by Cook County Hospital to the transferred patients at $3.35 million of which nearly $3 million was nonreimbursable; minimum costs that the private transferring hospitals would not have received had they provided care. Extrapolated for all of 1983, the total cost shifted to Cook County Hospital through transfers was $24 million.

Himmelstein, Woolhandler, and Harnly (1984), in a study of 458 patients transferred to the emergency department of Highland General Hospital in Oakland, California, found that about 63% had no insurance, 21% had Medicaid, and only 3% had private insurance. The study also found that a disproportionate number of transferred patients were minorities. Schiff et al. (1986) found that of 1,021 patient transfers to the Dallas Parkland Memorial Hospital, about 77% had no third-party insurance. The hospital spends some $10 million annually on transferred indigent patients (Frank, 1985). Ansell and Schiff (1987:1500) estimated that "250,000 patients nationwide in need of emergency care annually are transferred for economic reasons . . . representing a cost of 1.04 billion dollars to public hospitals."

Because hospitals are finding it increasingly difficult to shift the costs from one segment of their patient population to another, Ewe Reinhardt (1985:2) notes that "the uninsured poor themselves [have] become the hot potatoes one hospital seeks to dump into the lap of another." Until recently hospitals had little difficulty in shifting unreimbursed costs to essentially three other sources: private health insurance carriers and patients; charitable foundations and private donations; and private pay patients. With the decline in philanthropic donations hospitals only alternative in cost shifting has been the privately insured patient. These donations have in recent years covered no more than 4% of total health care costs (Milligan, 1986). In 1981 hospital cost shifting to private insured pay patients amounted to nearly $5 billion (Wehr, 1985). These costs are reflected in higher rates for employer sponsored health insurance through which a large number of individuals are insured. From 1977 to 1982 yearly payments by employers for health insurance benefits nationwide more than double from $33 billion to $78 billion (Berg, 1983). Recent cost containment strategies are reducing the hospitals' abilities to shift costs to the privately insured. With nowhere to shift the costs of unreimbursed care, hospitals, rather than absorb the costs, are dumping the uninsured individual.

Findings of some studies support the view that a primary reason for transfer is the inability of patients to pay. For example, research by Harvard Medical School doctors of 103 patients transferred from private hospitals to Highland General Hospital in Oakland, California showed not only that transfers jeopardized the patients in one-third of the cases but also that transfers were for economic reasons rather than patient care and "the transfers were a form of medical abuse" (Ansberry, 1988, 33).

EXPLANATIONS FOR HOSPITAL DUMPING

One explanation for the increase in dumping is that fewer patients have private hospital insurance. It is estimated that some 37 million people (15% of the total population) do not have medical insurance, Medicaid, or Medicare (Tolchin, 1988). An increase of some 8 million since 1979. This figure is growing at an alarming rate of 1 million individuals a year. About one-third are children under 18 years of age (Inglehart, 1985) and nearly 3 million are between the ages of 55 and 64 (Senator John Heinz, *Americans at Risk*, 1985:1). Another 50 million individuals are underinsured (Reinhardt, 1985).

The large numbers of uninsured and underinsured have caused hospitals, mostly public and voluntary not-for-profit hospitals, to provide $7.4 billion in uncompensated care in 1985. All total hospitals in 1985 provided $9.5 billion in free care (Brider, 1987). While dumping occurs in both urban and rural areas, it is most pronounced in large metropolitan areas, since this is where large numbers of uninsured are found.[2] In Chicago, for example, some 600,000 individuals (one of every five individuals) have no health insurance. In Illinois nearly 20% of the black and 25% of the Hispanic adult populations are uninsured (Marsh, 1988). Further, some 25% of the black population nationwide between the ages of 18 to 64 are uninsured (Bovbjerg and Kopit, 1986) and blacks represent about 17.3% or some 4 million of the total uninsured (Sulvetta and Swartz, 1986). Moreover, some 25% of all black children are uninsured and black children comprise some 20% or 2.2 million of all uninsured children under 18 years of age (Sulvetta and Swartz, 1986).

The dumping problem has been exacerbated by changes in Medicaid eligibility requirements which have increased the number of uninsured. President Reagan's budget pressures significantly reduced the number of individuals covered by Medicaid. In 1984 Medicaid covered only some 38% of the poor, compared with some 65% in 1976 (Brider, 1987).[3] With the enactment of the Omnibus Budget Reconciliation of 1981 (Public Law 97–35), Medicaid was reduced by some $12.8 billion mostly in federal matches to the states. In 1982 with the enactment of the Tax Equity and Fiscal Responsibilities Act (Public Law 97–248), Medicaid was reduced by another $2.2 billion through fiscal year 1985.

Private for-profit hospitals find it financially unattractive to provide care to the underinsured or to those unable to pay. As a result, private for-profit hospitals attempt to limit the number of uninsured patients they serve. Recent literature is supportive of this point. Rowland and Davis' (1982) analysis of the Office of Civil Rights (U.S. Department of Health and Human Services) survey data on inpatient admissions practices show that for-profit hospitals provided care to only 6% of uninsured patients in 1981. This compares to nearly 17% at state and local government hospitals. Their analysis also shows that of all the for-profit hospitals included in the survey data, about 60% had less than 5% uninsured admissions.

A second explanation has to do with the recent change in the way Medicare reimburses hospitals for care provided to elderly and disabled individuals.[4] Instead of reimbursing hospitals the actual costs of treating Medicare patients, the federal government now pays a set fee according to 467 "diagnostic-related groups" or DRGs (Social Security Act of 1983, Public Law 98-21). After a three-year phase-in period, by 1988 one national rate applied to all hospitals.

This new system, also referred to as a prospective payment system, has created a reverse effect on how hospitals treat and care for their patients (Pfeiffer and Christian, 1987). If a hospital spends less on a patient than the fixed reimbursed amount, it makes a profit. If the hospital spends more, it must absorb the loss. The incentive for hospitals then is to treat the elderly or disabled patient as economically and quickly as possible or not at all (Baldwin, 1985).

DRG abuses have been documented by several studies. A General Accounting Office study (1985) concludes that patients are being discharged from hospitals in poorer states of health. Guterman et al. (1988) report that the average length of stay for Medicare beneficiaries declined 9% during the first year of the system. Other studies report that the DRG system has led to increased transfers of Medicare patients to nursing homes and other extended care facilities with a greater level of debility at the time of transfer. Morrisey et al. (1988a), in an examination of patient discharge data from a national sample of 467 hospitals for the years 1980, 1983, 1984, and 1985, report that the proportion of Medicare patients transferred to post-hospital settings nearly doubled after implementation of the DRG System. Morrisey et al. (1988b) in a similar study of 501 hospitals, note that the prospective system increased the rate of discharges to subacute facilities.

Further, evidence now suggests that some hospitals will clearly be disadvantaged by the DRG system. These hospitals will tend to be those in rural areas (Mueller and Comer, 1987) and those with greater indigent and free care burdens (Valda, 1983; Aaron, 1984). Thus, the prospect exists that these hospitals may no longer be financially willing to provide care to those unable to pay or who are covered under the DRG system (Mueller and Comer, 1987). Thus it seems that increased dumping is directly related to the financial problems facing Medicaid/Medicare. Ironically, these two programs were enacted some 30 years ago to reduce the dumping of elderly and poor patients into charity wards and public hospitals.

A third explanation for an increase in dumping can be associated with the growing movement toward competitive health care, a reliance on market forces to determine the cost of care. While little empirical research has documented the effects competition has on costs and services of health care providers, it is quite clear that competition means hospitals are less likely to offer charity care. In the words of an administrator of a public hospital (cited in Millenson, 1987):

> To be medically indigent in a competitive system is tantamount
> to being an outcast [and] never in human history has economic
> competition resulted in the just distribution of scarce and life-
> sustaining resources.

Further, the competition strategy assumes that individuals can make informed decisions about hospital services. Yet, the medically indigent are the least likely to have the technical knowledge and varied experiences in medical care to make useful judgments about hospital care. This is especially so because of the limited health and hospital care providers available to the medically indigent. Moreover, emergency care for trauma or sudden illness for the medically indigent must be sought from the hospital willing or obligated to provide care, ruling out any possibility of a search.

HOSPITAL EMERGENCY CARE
AND THE MEDICALLY INDIGENT

In 1973 a court observed in *Mercy Medical Center* v. *Winnebago Co.* that:

> It would shock the public conscience if a person in need of
> emergency aid would be turned down at the door of a hospital
> having emergency service because that person could not at that
> moment assure payment for the service.

However, the traditional legal rule has been that hospitals are not required by "common law duty" to admit every person seeking admission.[5] This rule can be traced to a longstanding principle of tort law which holds that a person is not legally obligated to help another person in distress (Wing and Campbell, 1985). Under common law a hospital cannot be held liable for *nonfeasance*—for failure to render aid—to one in peril since it had no duty to act.[6] The Alabama Supreme Court in the 1934 case of *Birmingham Baptist Hospital* v. *Crews* in a seminal ruling held that a private hospital owes no duty to accept an emergency patient not desired by it and it does not have to provide a reason for refusal.[7]

In *Crews,* a two-year-old girl with diphtheria was provided initial treatment, denied further treatment, and sent home where she later died. Wing and Campbell (1985:130) equate the *Crews* ruling to a "drowning man" hypothetical:

> Assume a man is drowning in a lake with no hope of rescue. Must a passer-by who can easily throw a rope and save the man's life do so? The common-law answer is theoretically "no."

Using a similar analogy, Fine (1983) says:

> Like a competent swimmer who may let a child drown, . . . hospitals are under no legal duty to rescue . . .

The general rule (common law) in *Crews* has been maintained by courts in *Hill* v. *Ohio County* (1971), *LeJeune Road Hospital, Inc.* v. *Watson* (1965), and in *Harper* v. *Baptist Medical Center-Princeton* (1976). In *Hill,* a Kentucky court held that a public hospital had no duty to admit a pregnant woman who was about to give birth. In *Watson* a Florida District Court of Appeals ruled that a private hospital may reject any patient that it does not desire. In *Harper,* the Alabama Supreme Court reaffirmed its ruling in *Crews* by holding that the hospital was under no duty to admit the patient even after treating and stabilizing the patient in the emergency room.

However, the general rule established in *Crews* has been modified in several other court decisions. The courts have applied the concepts of "gratuitous undertaking" and "implied admission" to establish when a hospital is obligated to provide emergency care. The gratuitous undertaking theory imposes an obligation on the hospital once it begins to administer care. By beginning to render aid to an injured party, a hospital commits itself to providing emergency services to any member of the public in need of such services, assuming responsibility for the party's well-being and cannot discontinue service if it increases the risk of harm to the party (see Comment, 1974). Using the drowning man hypothetical in the gratuitous theory, Wing and Campbell (1985:130) make the following observation as applicable to *Crews*:

Assume that the passer-by undertakes to save the drowning man and throws a rope. Will the law obligate him to complete the effort, or may he arbitrarily abandon the rescue? . . . The reasoning [may be applied here] that [an] aborted rescue has not changed the drowning man's lot—he is still a drowning man, no better, no worse—so the passer-by has not *increased* the risk of harm.

A few decades later Prosser (cited in Wing and Campbell, 1985:131), using the same hypothetical, noted a change in reasoning and thus a change in liability:

It seems very unlikely that any court will ever hold that one who has began to pull a drowning man out of the river after he has caught hold of the rope, without good reason, to abandon the attempt, walk away, and let him drown, merely because he was already in extremis before the effort had begun.

The case of *O'Neill* v. *Montefiore Hospital* (1960) reflects this newer legal view of the gratuitous undertaking theory. In *O'Neill* the plaintiff entered the hospital room complaining of severe arm pains and believed he was having a heart attack. Montefiore Hospital did not accept patients with his kind of insurance policy. The attending nurse, however, did call a physician who worked with that kind of insurance. The plaintiff was instructed to go home until morning. Upon arriving home the plaintiff died of a heart attack. While there was no preexisting hospital/patient relationship, the court found the phone call made by the nurse could constitute a gratuitous undertaking.

The implied admission theory suggests that once a hospital begins treatment and care it has implicitly admitted the party and effectuated a hospital-patient contract (see Comment, 1974). Each of these theories require the performance of a specific act by a hospital which can be construed as an exercise of control over the patient. Court decisions in Mississippi (*New Biloxi Hospital, Inc.* v. *Frazier*, 1962), Tennessee (*Methodist Hospital* v. *Ball*, 1961), South Dakota (*Fjerstad* v. *Knutson*, 1978), and finally Florida (*Hunt* v. *Palm Springs General Hospital*, 1977) have advanced these theories. In *Frazier* (p. 197) the Mississippi Supreme Court outlined the hospital's duty to the patient:

In an emergency, the victim should be permitted to leave the hospital only after he has been seen, examined and offered reasonable first aid. In undertaking to do so, a hospital must exercise due care. A hospital emergency treatment is obligated to do that which is immediately and reasonably necessary for the preservation of the life, limb or health of the patient. I should not discharge a patient in critical condition without furnishing or procuring suitable medical attention.

In *Fjerstad* (pp. 11–12) the Supreme Court of South Dakota provided the following interpretation of the undertaking theory:

Although it has been held that a hospital, even one operating an emergency room, has no duty to accept a patient for treatment . . . once [a hospital] undertakes to render medical aid, the hospital is required to do so non-negligently. . . . The duty arose in this case, since the hospital undertook, through its nurses and intern, to render treatment to decedent. Decedent has a right to expect that the treatment rendered by a hospital which maintains and staffs an emergency room would be commensurate with that available in the same or similar communities or in hospitals generally.

While decisions in the more recent cases above may be viewed as favoring the medically indigent, the decisions in the earlier cases leaves the impact of case law on hospital behavior somewhat unclear. The decisions have not clearly established how and when patients status begins nor have they determined the criteria for hospital admission. On the one hand, the slightest undertaking on the part of the hospital can lead to a hospital-patient relationship. On the other hand, a hospital can flatly refuse to treat an individual and escape liability.

An alternate theory, used by several courts, holds a hospital liable for failure to render emergency care where an "unmistakable" emergency exists and the hospital has a well established custom of rendering emergency services (see *Wilmington General Hospital* v. *Manlove* 1961). Stated another way, this view, also known as the reliance theory (Dowell, 1984), holds that a hospital which maintains an emergency room is inviting for treatment patients who have a need for emergency care. The Delaware Supreme Court held in *Manlove* that the hospital may be liable even though treatment was not undertaken. Using this reasoning, the court avoided the problem of finding an affirmative act to trigger liability under the gratuitous undertaking and implied admission theories. Yet, the *Manlove* decision does not clearly point out hospital liability and duty to treat. In *Manlove* the court did not define when an "unmistaken emergency" exists, when a hospital has a "well-established custom of providing emergency care," and when prospective patient has a "reliance" on the hospital's custom of providing emergency care.

Defining Medical Emergency and Emergency Care

Until recently it was considered the social responsibility of a hospital to provide emergency care to those in need regardless of the ability to pay. In other words, to be treated in an emergency room for an emergency condition has been viewed as a secure nonstatutory right; that is, a right based on "the right to medical care" (Annas, 1986). Further, the public also considers the "emergency room as a neighborhood center, and expects it to provide around-the-clock primary care and emergency care with equal skill and speed" (Wing and Campbell, 1985:120). The general public definition of a medical emergency is "any illness or injury requiring immediate attention" (Dowell, 1984).

Similarly, national medical and physicians organizations also provide a broad definition of a medical emergency. The American Hospital Association (1982) defines an emergency

> as any condition that in the opinion of the patient, his family, or whoever assumes the responsibility of bringing the patient to the hospital requires immediate medical attention. This condition continues until a determination has been made by a health care professional that the patient's life or well-being is not threatened.

The American College of Surgeons has stated that "the function of an emergency department is to give adequate evaluation and initial treatment or advice to all persons who consider themselves acutely ill or injured and present themselves at the emergency room" (cited in Dowell, 1984). The American College of Emergency Physicians has defined a medical emergency as (cited in Dowell, 1984:484):

1. any condition resulting in admission of the patient to a hospital or nursing home within 24 hours;
2. evaluation or repair of acute (less than 72 hours) trauma;
3. relief of acute or severe pain;
4. investigation or relief of acute infection;
5. protection of public health;
6. obstetrical crises and/or labor;
7. hemorrhage or treatment of hemorrhage;
8. shock or impending shock; . . .
13. any sudden and/or serious symptom(s) which might indicate a condition which constitutes a threat to the patient's physical or psychological well being requiring immediate medical attention to prevent possible deterioration, disability, or death.

In some cases the courts have based their decisions on the emergency care policy provisions of national hospital and medical associations. In *Guerrero v. Copper Queen Hospital* (1975), the Arizona Court of Appeals relief on the emergency care provision of the Joint Commission on the Accreditation of Hospitals (1984) which states:

Any individual who comes to the hospital for emergency medical evaluation or initial treatment shall be properly assessed by qualified individuals and appropriate services shall be rendered within the defined capability of the hospital.

Individuals shall be accorded impartial access to treatment or accommodations that are available or medically indicated, regardless of race, creed, sex, national origin, or sources of payment of care.

In the *Guerrero* decision the court noted that:

If a hospital has been accredited by the Joint Commission on Hospital Accreditation, such Commission requires that its accredited hospital with emergency room facilities render emergency (care) to all who need it. It is arguable that by asking for a receiving accreditation, the hospital has undertaken a duty to the public, modifying the common law.

Further, the Arizona Court of Appeals held that the emergency treatment provision of the American Medical Association Code of Ethics obligates a physician to ensure that all patients are treated in the emergency room with the best of care.[4] These decisions seem to suggest that if there is a reasonable basis for suspecting that emergency care is necessary, a patient has a right to be examined and treated by a physician if the patient gets to the hospital emergency room.

The Emergency Transfer

It has also been legally established that a hospital's obligation to provide care continues even after the emergency condition has been stabilized until the patient is properly transferred or is medically fit for discharge (see, e.g., *Methodist Hospital* v. *Ball*, 1961). More recent decisions suggest that courts are likely to continue their view that public policy requires that emergency care be provided to those who need it (see, e.g., *St. Joseph's Hospital* v. *Maricopa Co.*, 1984). In *Thompson* the Arizona Supreme Court found the hospital liable for transferring a patient to the county hospital solely on economic grounds (see also Curran, 1985).

Although hospitals are within their legal rights to stabilize emergency patients and transfer them to other hospitals, they must do so in a nonnegligently and reasonable manner. A Louisiana Court addressed the "reasonableness" issue in *Joyner* v. *Alton Ochsner Medical Foundation* (1970) and ruled in favor of the hospital. In *Joyner* after providing initial emergency treatment, the hospital refused to admit the patient without a deposit and transferred him. The patient sued for pain and suffering incurred during the transfer.

Conversely, in *Jones* v. *City of New York Hospital for Joint Diseases* (1954), the New York Supreme Court found the hospital liable for transferring a patient without rendering emergency surgery. In another case, a Pennsylvania Supreme Court in *Riddle Memorial Hospital* v. *Dohan* (1984), reaffirmed the lower court's decision that the hospital had acted in a reasonable manner in allowing the patient to be transferred. An interesting aspect of this case was that the patient's private physician was the attending physician at Riddle and favored the transfer to another hospital.

Despite the present legal standards requiring hospitals to provide emergency care to those who need it, the increased emphasis on cost containment is transforming medical care from a social good to an economic one. Not only has the rise of for-profit hospitals challenged the traditional social commitment of hospitals to provide emergency services to the uninsured and poor, but so has the lessening of the social commitment on the part of government itself. The government's emphasis on cost containment has made quality of care and equity of access concerns secondary issues (Greensberg, 1984). This new economics of medicine means a fierce competition among hospitals that must keep one eye on healing and the other on the bottom line. Providing hospital care to the medically indigent and the poor has become an intolerable expense on the part of many hospitals.

In fact, some hospitals have closed completely or have chosen not to provide emergency care because of the financial situation created by medical indigency problems. In Los Angeles the problem of uncompensated care was a contributing factor in the closing of 11 hospitals in the area since 1985 (Brider, 1987). Several other hospitals have chosen to discontinue their participation in the Los Angeles area's trauma network because of the increasing number of uninsured trauma patients (Brider, 1987). Still other hospitals have downgraded their emergency rooms to avoid having to accept uninsured emergency trauma cases (Brom, 1986). These situations, coupled with the nationwide increase in the closures of private for-profit hospitals and public hospitals in the inner city (Rice, 1987), are making it increasingly difficult for the medically indigent to locate a source of hospital care.

PUBLIC POLICY RESPONSE TO DUMPING

Texas became the first state to effect comprehensive regulations that specifically deal with the dumping problem. The regulations which are mandated by Texas law and were promulgated by the Texas State Board of Health became effective in April 1986. The regulations prohibit dumping of emergency patients and ensure that patients are transferred only with their informed consent (when possible) and for valid medical reasons (Relman, 1986). The regulations also require hospitals to submit a transfer policy to the Texas Department of Health. A hospital not submitting an acceptable policy by a specified time risks losing its license to operate and being fined not more than $1,000 for each act of violation. The legislation was provided impetus by Parkland Memorial Hospital in Dallas which effectuated a policy and study of patient transfers in 1983 (Reed, Cawley, and Anderson, 1986).

Further, in 1983 the Texas legislature enacted a law making hospitals and physicians liable for felony prosecutions if they denied medical care to individuals because of socioeconomic considerations (Berg, 1983). At the time of the legislation, Texas ranked forty-eighth among the states in the level of payments to hospitals for the poor (Berg, 1983). New York in 1983 passed a statute that made economic emergency refusals a misdemeanor punishable by a fine of $1,000 and a year in jail for the hospital personnel involved. The State of New York may also revoke a hospital's operating license for denying emergency care after a judicial hearing. In June 1985, South Carolina enacted an antidumping law which included a civil penalty of up to $10,000 if violated by a hospital (Dallek and Waxman, 1986).

Some 25 states have enacted legislation requiring hospitals to provide emergency care regardless of ability to pay and requiring that patients be stabilized before transfer (Ansell and Schiff, 1987). However, many of the state statutes are ineffective and are rarely enforced. Treiger (1986:1186) notes that "the central weakness of most state statutes is that they do not contain a clear definition of emergency services" and those states which have remedies, have weak ones. For example, Georgia and South Carolina fines range from $100 to $500 for violating hospitals (Treiger, 1986). At the local government level, Alameda County and Los Angeles County, California, have developed a set of guidelines for hospital transfers (Comment, 1974).

At the federal level, the Consolidated Omnibus Budget Reconciliation Act (COBRA) enacted by Congress in 1985 (Public Law 99-272) prohibits patient dumping. The law requires hospitals to provide a medical examination and the necessary treatment to stabilize the condition of anyone who comes to the hospital with severe, acute symptoms (Parks and Dallek, 1986). A hospital or physician found in violation of this requirement is subject to a civil penalty of up to $25,000 per case. Brookside Hospital, a public hospital in San Pablo, California, became the first facility to face fines and sanctions under the law. The U.S. Department of Health and Human Services (DHHS) began investigating five cases of alleged patient dumping at the hospital. If found in violation, the hospital would not only be subject to civil penalty as is prescribed by law but also could be denied its Medicare/Medicaid reimbursements which in 1986 amounted to nearly $25 million. The legislation also requires that if an emergency exists, a hospital must stabilize or transfer the patient to a facility that can; and a hospital cannot transfer an unstable patient unless another facility can offer better treatment (Burda, 1987).

By late 1987, DHHS had received only 33 complaints of patient dumping. Table 7.1 provides a listing of complaints filed with DHHS as of October 1987. More than 50% of the complaints came from the state of Texas. Only five actions had been taken against hospitals. A most prominent hospital charged with dumping was the University of Chicago Hospital where there occurred an allegedly illegal transfer of a gunshot victim in July 1987. DHHS issued termination of Medicare participation against the hospital. After adding a trauma team and promising such an incident would not occur again, the facility was exonerated. By January 31, 1988, DHHS had received 129 complaints, and fines had been levied and Medicare termination disqualification had been initiated against only two hospitals. By mid-1988, DHHS had received 188 complaints alleging patient dumping, and 53 were found not to have complied with the law (Tolchin, 1988). By late 1988, 61 hospitals were found by DHHS to have violated the antidumping law (Ansberry, 1988).

Despite the increase in antidumping legislation at the state and federal government levels, several shortcomings have become evident and need to be addressed. First, legislation needs to provide mechanism(s) for monitoring and enforcement/compliance. Second, legislation needs to define more clearly and precisely what a medical emergency is and what it means to stabilize a person before transfer (see Ansell and Schiff, 1987). Defining stabilization is most

TABLE 7.1. Hospital Dumping Complaints Filed with DHHS*

Region	Date Complaint Received	Name of Hospital	Section of COBRA Alleged Noncompliance	In Progress	In Compliance	Out of Compliance
III	01/16/87	Mary Washington Fredericksburg, VA	Treatment and transfer for active labor	X		
IV	04/27/87	Methodist, Somerville, IN	Stabilizing treatment, transfer	X		
	12/04/87	Jennie Stuart Hopkinsville, KY	Stabilizing treatment, transfer	X		
	01/08/87	Marymount, London, KY	Stabilizing treatment		X	
	01/27/87	George County/Mobile Lucedale, MS	Treatment, transfer for active labor		X	
	02/24/87	Goodlark, Dickson, TN	Stabilizing treatment		X	
	04/08/87	Jackson-Madison, Jackson, TN	Stabilizing treatment	X		
	04/01/87	Methodist Evangelical Louisville, KY	Treatment, transfer	X		
VI	01/05/87	Humana, Clear Lake, TX	Stabilizing treatment, transfer	X		
	01/06/87	Dermot-Chicot Dermot, TX	Screening, treatment, transfer active labor	X		
	04/08/87	South Plains Amherst, TX	Treatment, transfer	X		

*As of October 9, 1987.

TABLE 7.1 (continued)

Region	Date Complaint Received	Name of Hospital	Section of COBRA Alleged Noncompliance	In Progress	In Compliance	Out of Compliance
	05/05/87	Fannin County, Bonham, TX	Treatment, transfer	X		
	05/05/87	Lillian, Sonora, TX	Treatment, transfer	X		
	05/05/87	Wintergarden Memorial Dilly, TX	Treatment, transfer	X	(termination underway)	
	05/05/87	Charter Community Cleveland, TX	Treatment, transfer			X
	05/12/87	Trinity Memorial Trinity, TX	Treatment, transfer	X		
	05/12/87	Riverside Corpus Christi, TX	Treatment, transfer	X		
	05/12/87	Terrell Community Terrell, TX	Treatment, transfer	X		
	5/12/87	San Saba, San Saba, TX	Treatment, transfer	X		
	05/12/87	Mitchell County Colorado City, TX	Treatment, transfer	X		
	05/12/87	South Arlington Medical Center, Arlington, TX	Treatment, transfer	X		
	05/27/87	Oakgrove Louisiana West Carroll Parish, LA	Treatment, transfer	X		
	05/27/87	Central Texas Memorial Center, Hearne, TX	Treatment, transfer	X		

TABLE 7.1 (continued)

Region	Date Complaint Received	Name of Hospital	Section of COBRA Alleged Noncompliance	In Progress	In Compliance	Out of Compliance
	04/15/87	Trinity Memorial Trinity, TX	Treatment, transfer	X		
	12/30/86	Lewisville Medical Lewisville, TX	Treatment	X		
	01/28/87	McAllen Medical McAllen, TX	Refuse to accept indigent transfers		X	
	02/17/87	Detar, Victoria, TX	Treatment transfer for active labor	X		
	02/20/87	Alvin Community Alvin, TX	Treatment, transfer		X	
	11/21/86	HCA Valley Brownsville, TX	Treatment, transfer		X	
	04/01/87	Colonial, Terrell, TX	Treatment, transfer		X	
	04/01/87	Wilson N. Jones Sherman, TX	Screening, treatment, transfer		X	
	03/18/87	Brookside, San Pablo, TX	Treatment, transfer	(termination rescinded)		X
IX	04/09/87	Los Medanos Pittsburg, CA	Transfer	X		

Source: Committee on Government Operations, *Equal Access to Health Care: Patient Dumping,* Hearing Before a Subcommittee on Government Operations, House of Representatives, 100th Congress, 1st Session, July 22, 1987 (Washington, DC: Government Printing Office, 1988), pp. 210–211.

important because as Relman (1986:373) points out "'stabilization' of emergency cases is a notion used by hospital managers to justify transfers for economic reasons, but it is an elusive and dangerous concept." In other words, present legislation as written may still allow patients' conditions to be misrepresented in private hospitals' efforts to transfer them to public hospitals.

Third, the legislation needs to address more closely the medical aspects of patient dumping. The point here is that patients in need of emergency care are being denied appropriate care and treatment. Studies (Himmelstein, Woolhandler, and Harnly, 1984; Anderson, Cowley, and Andrulis, 1984; Schiff et al., 1986; and Wrenn, 1985) have shown and reports by the popular media have noted (Okie, 1986) that transfers have jeopardized the patients' well-being because of delayed treatments or lack of treatments. The transfer also leads to problems in testing and lab procedures duplication (Hicks et al., 1986) and increased pain and suffering on the part of the transferred patients (Ansell and Schiff, 1987).

In response to these concerns, the Health Care Financing Administration in DHHS, the agency charged with enforcement, proposed new antidumping regulations. Congress adopted the regulations as an amendment to COBRA in April 1986. The regulations become effective on August 1, 1987. The gist of the regulations are: (1) when pregnant patients are in active labor, they cannot be transferred; (2) a hospital cannot transfer a patient unless his or her medical condition has been stabilized; (3) a transfer can take place if a doctor certifies in writing that the transfer to the receiving hospital outweighs the risk of transfer if better treatment is available. The regulations define stabilize as "providing medical treatment of the condition necessary to assure, within reasonable medical probability, that no material deterioration of the condition is likely to result from the transfer." Congress increased the civil monetary penalty from $25,000 to $50,000 (U.S. House of Representatives 3545 Conference Report, 1987).

Despite these changes, the legislation needs to be amended with additional provisions. First, the legislation needs to require that a *memo of transfer* be signed by the sending hospital physician and the receiving hospital physician. This process would serve initially to document the transfer through written record, and then to place accountability on physicians, particularly the transferring physician, regarding the patient's health and the dumping provision. Second, the legislation needs to require a posted notice in hospitals about the law. Hill-Burton hospitals are required by DHHS to post notices concerning their Hill-Burton obligations (Rice and Jones, 1985). This provision would help make the law more knowledgeable to individuals and would perhaps increase compliance.

CONCLUSION

Hospitals whether public or private (for-profit) exist to serve the needs of patients. Yet present government policy seems to be telling hospitals that they must become more cost conscious, that is, act like competitive businesses. In this kind of climate, hospital care for the indigent and the uninsured is not a very high concern particularly for private for-profit hospitals. As Relman (1985:372) observes, "When business considerations dominate the behavior of hospital management, the poor will be inevitably neglected." Patient dumping may be viewed as a most serious form of neglect.

While public policy is now addressing the patient dumping problem at the federal level and in some state and local laws, more comprehensive laws and court decisions are also needed that require all hospitals, regardless of ownership, to treat all emergency patients who arrive at their doors if the hospitals have the appropriate medical staff and facilities. Less than half of the states have enacted statutes concerning emergency medical care or health care for those without insurance. If economic rather than medical reasons continue to be the motivation for patient dumping for hospitals not to provide care, then individuals will continue to be at high risk of not receiving necessary hospital care. This will especially be the case for the black community.

NOTES

1. The four largest private profit making hospital chains, Hospital Corporation of America, Humana, Inc., American Medical International, and National Medical Enterprises, earned $297 million, $193 million, $155 million and $127 million, respectively, in 1984 (see Kraft, 1985).

2. The largest percentage of the total uninsured are found in the West South Central and Mountain geographical regions in the United States with 20.2% and

19.2% respectively. The New England and Middle Atlantic regions have the smallest percentage of the total uninsured with 10.5% and 12.5%, respectively (see Sulvetta and Swartz, 1986).

3. About 23 million low income individuals were covered by Medicaid in fiscal year 1986 (see Treiger, 1986, note 18).

4. Some 29 million aged and 3 million disabled individuals are covered under Medicare (see Treiger, 1986, note 18).

5. A similar ruling applicable to doctors can be traced to the Indiana Supreme Court in *Hurley* v. *Eddingfield* (1901).

6. Nonfeasance is unlike malfeasance, which is an affirmative act causing injury or increased risk of harm to another. Malfeasance imposes a duty to provide aid.

7. A Georgia Court of Appeals has ruled that a *public* hospital that maintains emergency facilities open to the general public cannot arbitrarily refuse to provide emergency services to any member of the public in need of such services.

REFERENCES

Aaron, H.J. (1984). "Prospective Payment: The Next Disappointment?" *Health Affairs* (Fall):102–107.

American Hospital Association (1982). *Hospital Terminology.* Chicago, IL: American Hospital Association Press.

Americans at Risk: The Case of the Medically Uninsured. Hearings Before the Senate Special Committee on Aging (1985), 99th Congress, 1st Session.

Anderson, R.J., Cowley, K.A., and Andrulis, D.P. (1984). "The Evolution of a Public Hospital Transfer Policy." Paper presented at the 112th Annual Meeting of the American Public Health Association. Anaheim, CA, November 13.

Annas, G.J. (1986). "Your Money or Your Life: 'Dumping' Uninsured Patients from Hospital Emergency Wards." *American Journal of Public Health* (January):74–77.

Ansberry, C. (1988). "Dumping the Poor: Despite Federal Law, Hospitals Still Reject Sick Who Can't Pay." *Wall Street Journal* (November 29):A1, A10.

Ansell, D.A., and Schiff, R.L. (1987). "Patient Dumping: Status, Implications and Policy Recommendations." *Journal of the American Medical Association* 257 (March 20):1500–1502.

Baldwin, M.F. (1985). "Lawmakers Focus on Hospital DRG Squeeze." *Modern Healthcare* (March):54–58.

Berg, T. (1983). "Major Corporations Ask Workers to Pay More of Health Care." *New York Times* (September 12):A1.

Bishop, K. (1987). "Hospital May Lose Funds Over Transfers of Poor." *New York Times* (April 1).

Bovbjerg, R.R., and Kopit. W.G. (1986). "Coverage and Care for the Medically Indigent: Public and Private Options." *Indiana Law Review* 19:857–917.

Brider, P. (1987). "Too Poor To Pay: The Scandal of Patient Dumping." *American Journal of Nursing* (November):1447–1449.

Brom, T. (1986). "Death By a Thousand Cuts." *California Lawyer* 6 (April):19–20.

Burda, D. (1987). "Dumping Law Spurs Look at E D Risk Management." *Hospitals* (July 20):34–38.

"Checking the Patients Before His Credit." (Editorial) (1986). *The Atlanta Constitution* (April 1):A-14.

Comment (1974). "Liability of Private Hospital Emergency Rooms for Refusal to Provide Emergency Care." *Mississippi Law Journal* 45:1003–1028.

Curran, W.J. (1985). "Law-Medicine Notes: Economic and Legal Considerations in Emergency Care." *New England Journal of Medicine* (February 7):374–375.

Dallek, G. (1983). "For-Profit Hospitals and the Poor." *Clearinghouse Review* (December):860–867.

Dallek, G., and Waxman, J. (1986). "Patient Dumping: A Crisis in Emergency Medical Care for the Indigent." *Clearinghouse Review* (April):1413–1417.

Dowell, M.A. (1984). "Indigent Access to Hospital Emergency Room Services." *Clearinghouse Review* (October 1984):483–492.

Duncan, R.P., and Vogel, W.B. (1988). "Uncompensated Care and the Inpatient Transfer." Presented at the Annual Meeting of the American Public Health Association. Boston, MA.

Editorial (1982). "Hospitals Said 'No.'" *Des Moines Register* (May 18).

Ellis, V. (1985). "Compromise Paves Way for Outlining 'Patient Dumping'." *Dallas Times Herald* (December 13).

"15% of Transfers Seen as 'Dumping'" (1986). *Hospitals* (October 5):146.

Fine, J. E. (1983). "Opening the Closed Doors: The Duty of Hospitals to Treat Emergency Room Patients." *Washington Journal of Urban and Contemporary Law* 24:123–150.

Frank, C. (1985). "Dumping the Poor: Private Hospitals Risk Suits." *American Bar Association Journal* 71 (March):25.

Friedman, E. (1982). "Special Report—The Dumping Dilemma: Finding What's Fair." *Hospitals* (September 18):75–84.

General Accounting Office (1985). *Medicare: PPS Impact on Post-Hospital Long-Term Care Services* (Washington, DC: GAO/PEMO-85-8, February 21).

Greensberg, D.S. (1984). "Health Care Thrift Spurs Patient Dumping." *Los Angeles Times* (November 12).

Guterman, S., Eggers, P., Riley, G., Greene, T., and Terrell, S. (1988). "The First Three Years of Medicare Prospective Payment: An Overview." *Health Care Financing Review* 9(3):67-77.

Hicks, T.C., Danzl, D.F., Thomas, D.M. et al. (1986). "Resuscitation and Transfer of Trauma Patients: A Prospective Study." *Annals of Emergency Medicine*, 296–299.

"Hospital Rejected Women in Labor, May Lose Funds." (1986) *The Atlanta Constitution* (October 2):A-8.

Himmelstein, D.U., Woolhandler, S., and Harnly, M. (1984). "Patient Transfer: Medical Practice as Social Triage." *American Journal of Public Health* 74:494–497.

"Hospitals in Cost Squeeze 'Dump' More Patients Who Can't Pay Bills" (1985). *The Wall Street Journal* (March 8).

Inglehart, J.K. (1985). "Medical Care of the Poor: A Growing Problem." *New England Journal of Medicine* (January):59–63.

Joint Commission on the Accreditation of Hospitals (1984). *Accreditation Manual of Hospitals*, 1985 ed.: (Chicago: Joint Commission on the Accreditation of Hospitals).

Klaidman, D. (1986). "D.C. General: Hospital or Dumping Ground?" *Washington Post* (December 29).

Kraft, J. (1985). "Hospitals for Profit: What Price Care?" *Los Angeles Times* (March 31):1,33.

Marsh, B. (1988). "The Medical Indigence Crisis." *Crain's Chicago Business,* 11 (43) (October 24):1,100–104.

"Medicare DRGs Pose Problems for the Elderly" (1985). *Hospitals* (December 16):75–76.

Millenson, M. (1987). "The Unhealthy Medical Care of the Poor." *Business and Society Review* (Spring):40–43.

Milligan, C.J., Jr. (1986). "Provisions of Uncompensated Care in American Hospitals: The Role of Tax Code, The Federal Courts, Catholic Health Care Facilities, and Local Government in Defining the Problem of Access for the Poor." *Catholic Lawyer* 31 (1):7–34.

Morrisey, M.A. et al. (1988a). "Post Hospitals Transfers Under Medicare Prospective Payment." *Health Affairs*. (In Press).

Morrisey, M.A. et al. (1988b). "Medicare Prospective Payment and Posthospital Transfers to Subacute Care." *Medicare Care 26*(7) (July):685–698.

Mueller, K.J., and Comer, J.C. (1987). "Providers' Predictions of Effects of the Prospective Payment System." *Journal of Health and Human Resources Administration* (Fall 1987):147–155.

Okie, S. (1986). "'Dumping' Patients into Public Hospitals May Shorten Lives, Study Says." *The Washington Post* (February 27):A-14.

Parks, M.C., and Dallek, G. (1986). "New COBRA Legislation Adopts Many Changes in Medicare and Other Health Programs." *Clearinghouse Review* (August/September):562–572.

"Patient 'Dumping' Regulations Offer Little Guidance" (1987). *Hospitals* (September 5):35–36.

Perkins, J. et al. (1986). "State Based Financing of Indigent Health Care: Promise and Problems." *Clearinghouse Review* Special Issue (Summer 1986):372–381.

Pfeiffer, D., and Christian, P. (1987). "Impact of the Federal Prospective Payment System Upon Long-Term Care Related Medicare Patients." *Journal of Health and Human Resources Administration* (Fall):115–146.

Reed, W.G., Cawley, K.A., and Anderson, R.J. (1986). "Special Report: The Effect of a Public Hospital's Transfer Policy on Patient Care." *New England Journal of Medicine* (November 27):1428–1432.

Reinhardt, E. (1985). "Editorial: Health and Hot Potatoes." *The Washington Post* (March 16):2.

Relman, A.S. (1985). "Economic Considerations In Emergency Care: What Are Hospitals For?" *New England Journal of Medicine* (February 7):372–373.

Relman, A.S. (1986). "Texas Eliminates Dumping: A Start Toward Equity in Hospital Care." *New England Journal of Medicine* (February 27):578–579.

Rice, M.F. (1985/86). "The Urban Public Hospital: Its Importance to the Black Community." *Urban League Review* 9(2) (Winter):64–70.

Rice, M.F. (1987). "Inner-City Hospital Closures/Relocations: Race, Income Status and Legal Issues." *Social Science and Medicine* 24(11):889–896.

Rice, M.F., and Jones, Jr., W. (1985). "Public Policy and Black Health Care: A Civil Rights Perspective." In M.D. Tryman (ed.), *Institutional Racism and Black America* (Lexington, MA: Ginn Press):67–99.

Rowland, D., and Davis, K. (1982). "The Uninsured and Inpatient Hospital Care." Paper Presentation at the 110th Annual Meeting of the American Public Association Annual Meeting. Montreal, Canada, November.

Schiff, R.L., Ansell, D.A., Schlosser, J.E., Idris, A.H., Morrison, A., and Whitman, S. (1986). "Transfers to a Public Hospital: A Prospective Study of 467 Patients." *New England Journal of Medicine* (February 27):552–557.

Segar, A. (1983). "The Reconfiguration of Urban Hospital Care." In A.L. Green and S. Green (eds.), *Cities and Sickness: Health Care in Urban America* (Beverly Hills: Sage Publications).

"Senior Citizens Seek Protection" (1986). *The Boston Globe* (November 2):53.

Sulvetta, M.B., and Swartz, K. (1986). *The Uninsured and Uncompensated Care: A Chartbook* (Washington, DC: National Health Policy Forum).

"TDH Rules on Hospital Transfers Take Effect April 1" (1986). *Texas Medicine* 82 (March):59–62.

"The New World of Health Care" (1986). *U.S. News and World Report* (April 14):60–63.

Tolchin, M. (1988). "U.S. Seeks to Require Treatment of All Hospital Emergency Cases." *The New York Times* (June 18):1, 8.

Treiger, K.I. (1986). "Preventing Patient Dumping: Sharpening the COBRA's Fangs." *New York University Law Review* 61 (December):1186–1223.

U.S. House of Representatives (1987). *Omnibus Budget Reconciliation Act of 1987: Conference Report to Accompany H.R. 3545* (Washington, DC: Government Printing Office, December 21, 1987).

Valda, M.I. (1983). "The Financial Impact of Prospective Payment on Hospitals." *Health Affairs* (Spring):112–119.

Wehr, B. (1985). "Hospitals, Insurers, Patients Feeling Pinch of Federal Cutbacks in Medicare, Medicaid Funds," *Congressional Quarterly Weekly Report* (July 17).

Wing, K.R., and Campbell, J.R. (1985). "The Emergency Room Admission: How Far Does the 'Open Door' Go?" *University of Detroit Law Review* 63:119–144.

Wrenn, K. (1985). "Sounding Board: No Insurance, No Admission." *New England Journal of Medicine* (February 7):373–374.

COURT CASES

Birmingham Baptist Hospital v. *Crews*, 157 Ala. So. 224 (1934).

Fjerstad v. *Knutson*, 271 N.W. 2d 8 (S.D. 1978).

Guerrero v. *Copper Queen Hospital*, 112 Ariz. 104, 537 P.2d 1329 (1975).

Harper v. *Baptist Medical Center–Princeton*, 341 So. 2d 133 (Ala, 1976).

Hill v. *Ohio County*, 468 S.W. 2d 306 (Ky. 1971).

Hunt v. *Palm Springs General Hospital*, 352 So. 2d 582 (Fla. 1977).

Hurley v. *Eddingfield*, 156 Ind. 416, 59 N.E. 1058 (1901).

Jones v. *City of New York Hospital for Joint Diseases*, 134 N.Y.S. 2d 779 (Sup.Ct. 1954).

Joyner v. *Alton Ochsner Medical Foundation*, 230 So. 2d 913 (La.Ct.App. 1970).

LeJeune Road Hospital, Inc. v. *Watson*, 171 So. 2d 202 (Fla.Dist.Ct.App. 1965).

Mercy Medical Center v. *Winnebago Co.*, 206 N.W. 2d 198 (Wisc. 1973).

Methodist Hospital v. *Ball*, 50 Tenn. App. 460, 362 S.W. 2d 475 (1961).

New Biloxi Hospital, Inc. v. *Frazier*, 146 Miss. So. 2d (1962).

O'Neill v. *Montefiore Hospital*, 202 N.Y.S. 2d 436 (1960).

Riddle Memorial Hospital v. *Dohan*, 504 Pa. 571, 475 A. 2d 1314 (1984).

St. Joseph's Hospital v. *Maricopa Co.*, 688 Ariz. P.2d 605 (1984).

Wilmington General Hospital v. *Manlove*, 54 Del. 15, 174 A.2d 135 (1961).

Chapter 8

A Programmatic Approach to Improving the Health of Poor Children

Valire Carr Copeland

There is a consensus among policy makers, physicians, child health advocates, and the general public on the need for federal action to improve health care services for poor children in the United States. The National Governors Association, several bipartisan groups, and others concerned with the health status of the nation's poor children are calling for sweeping reforms in the health care system. What should be done, how it will be done, and who should be responsible remain controversies.

Progress toward improving the health of children, especially those who are poor, has slowed (American Academy of Pediatrics, 1989; Hill and Breyel, 1991; Klerman, 1991; National Commission on Children, 1991; National Center for Children in Poverty, 1990; Sardell, 1990). The percentage of low birthweight births has not decreased since 1980; immunization rates among children have declined while the incidence of measles, mumps, and rubella has increased; and the number of children in poverty has increased and this increase is expected to continue. The correlation between poverty and poor health is evidenced by children's lack of financial access to health care; an estimated 12 million children, mostly poor children, are at risk for lead poisoning; and of the more than 33 million Americans without health insurance, one-third are children (National Commission on Children (NCC), 1991).

This chapter was previously published in *Journal of Health & Social Policy*, Vol. 6(4) 1995.

Since 1984, federal and state governments have provided additional resources for designing and implementing programs to reduce the infant mortality rate in this country. Title XIX and Title V program officials have worked together to improve the access and quality of publicly funded prenatal care programs for poor pregnant women. Unfortunately, the focus on pregnant women and their unborn children has not stimulated the same level of enthusiasm on behalf of poor children over six years of age (Hill and Breyel, 1991). Moreover, in 1990 we witnessed a decrease in the nation's infant mortality rate, but 9.1 deaths per 1,000 births is still higher than 21 other industrialized nations. African-American babies are still twice as likely to die as white babies (NCC, 1991), and the percentage of low-birthweight babies for African-American women has increased. Despite the more obvious improvements, the health problems of poor children at risk persist, and other problems, such as prenatal exposure to dangerous drugs and AIDS, have emerged (National Commission to Prevent Infant Mortality, 1990). Poor children are at a greater risk than nonpoor children for developing chronic and disabling conditions. They are also confronted with other health and developmental problems that can prevent them from being productive members of society in adulthood. A comprehensive child health care program can provide services that will help poor children develop into healthy adults, prevent chronic disabling conditions, and save money by having more productive adults in the workforce in later years.

There is a longstanding program that might, if expanded and better implemented, do the job—the Early and Periodic Screening Diagnosis and Treatment (EPSDT) program. Because EPSDT offers an array of screening, diagnostic, and follow-up services to prevent the onset of chronic disabling conditions and covers both physical and mental health problems, it has the greatest potential of all extant programs for improving the delivery of health care services to poor children. But due to the lack of enthusiasm for the program in many states, the carelessness of the way in which it was implemented, the low enrollment of eligible recipients, and the low rates of provider participation, the program has not lived up to its potential (Foltz, 1975; Hill and Breyel, 1991; Klerman, 1991). For EPSDT to function effectively, it should be separated from the welfare bureaucracy and reassembled in the health bureaucracy, nationally. The strategy suggested in this chapter would require state officials to restructure EPSDT and integrate it with other Maternal and Child Health (MCH) services programs. This chapter addresses the problems and potential of EPSDT within the context of Medicaid—since EPSDT is a part of Medicaid, it is difficult to examine the nature of the problems that plague EPSDT without also discussing Medicaid—and proposes a programmatic strategy to make EPSDT more effective.

EPSDT AND MATERNAL AND CHILD HEALTH SERVICES: AN OVERVIEW

The health services provided by EPSDT are very similar to some of the child health services provided by the Maternal and Child Health services programs (Hanlon and Pickett, 1984; Carr, 1989; Klerman, 1991; Department of Health and Human Services (DHHS), 1990). Both MCH services and EPSDT programs provide primary and preventive child health services to poor children which include: screening, diagnosis, and treatment services for medical, visual, hearing, and dental ailments; health care for adolescents; care for high-risk infants, children, and youth; and immunizations. However, MCH services programs offer a wider selection of additional programs for maternal and child populations. MCH service offerings go beyond those provided by EPSDT. MCH programs are administered by state health agencies and, in the majority of states, EPSDT programs are administered by state welfare agencies. Throughout EPSDT's tenure, Congress has repeatedly recommended that Title XIX officials and Title V officials work together to coordinate the delivery of child health services. In its report, the Select Panel for the Promotion of Child Health (DHHS, 1981), recommended that each state be urged to consolidate the functions of its child health programs under one agency. In some states this has happened; in others it has not.

When EPSDT was initially formulated in 1967, it was viewed as a blueprint for a national health care program for all poor children. The program was designed to provide comprehensive health care services to all poor children. As an incremental adjustment to the Medicaid legislation, the EPSDT provisions required states to establish a primary and preventive child health services delivery system for Medicaid eligible children. According to Sardell (1990), the EPSDT program was to be structured to bring together all child health services. This has not happened. EPSDT is unique because the health service provisions are mandated: (1) to educate families and their children about the value of health care, (2) to provide periodic visual, hearing, dental, and health care screening, (3) to diagnose and assess the severity of any health problem discovered during screening, and (4) to provide the health care that is needed to ameliorate the diagnosed illness and prevent acute ailments from becoming chronic crippling conditions. EPSDT was the first federal government program that required state officials "to reach out and bring poor children into care even if their parents had not sought it" (Klerman, 1991, p. 13).

The next five sections of this chapter present the following: a chronology of the EPSDT program and the legislative changes that have strengthened it as a major source of health care for selected poor children; a focus on the state participation rates of eligible children with emphasis on the low enrollments as indicators of how poorly the programs are performing; a discussion of low provider participation as an obstacle to care for Medicaid recipients and the financial and other issues faced when providing care; an examination of how EPSDT could be administered to enhance its effectiveness by addressing the controversy over whether EPSDT should be administered by state welfare or state health agencies; and an examination of how EPSDT has improved the health of some poor children and argument that EPSDT should be integrated with state MCH services programs. I conclude that restructuring EPSDT will provide the comprehensive program that was desired when EPSDT was conceived, and that this restructuring strategy may be a more viable solution to the crisis in child health given the absence of an acceptable national reform policy.

EPSDT—THE FEDERAL RESPONSE

One of the issues that plagued the EPSDT program from its inception was the fact that Congress could never decide whether EPSDT was a health or a welfare program. Attaching the program to Medicaid stigmatized it as a welfare program. However, its chronology over the years clearly validates it as a child health program that is primarily administered in a welfare bureaucracy. Since EPSDT is a Medicaid program, any changes in Medicaid affect EPSDT. Under Public Law 90-248, the 1967 amendments to the Social Security Act, Title XIX programs are mandated to provide early and periodic screening, diagnosis, and treatment services to eligible children under 21 years of age. Provisions for encouraging early case findings of defects and chronic illnesses of children and for remedying these defects were legislated.[1]

Over the years, Congress has legislated other changes that strengthen EPSDT as a comprehensive child health program. Some of these changes have helped, but others have limited the extent to which EPDST can fulfill its promise. When state officials were resistant to the EPSDT mandate and slow to implement the program, Congress enacted a penalty amendment to penalize states that failed to comply with the mandate. Several states were found out of compliance, but the penalty was never enforced. The penalty amendment was later removed through the Omnibus Budget Reconciliation Act (OBRA) of 1981. In 1985, Congress required EPSDT benefits to be consistent with established medical and dental standards. State program officials are required to enroll eligible children in continuing care arrangements and to encourage more coordinated comprehensive care.

The 1989 expansion provisions of OBRA for EPSDT have been the most significant in expanding eligibility and strengthening the service components of the program since its inception. As a result of this act, states must provide health education of children and advise parents about the EPSDT screening examination. Federal rules for provider participation are clarified so that a larger pool of providers can be qualified to provide EPSDT screening examinations. New annual state reporting requirements are mandated. Together with the Secretary of Health and Human Services, state officials have set goals for annual participation rates for EPSDT programs nationwide (Sardell, 1990; Klerman, 1991; Hill and Breyel, 1991; DHHS, 1988; Bergman, 1990; National Center for Clinical Infant Programs, 1990). Hill and Breyel (1991) anticipated that by 1995, 80% of the eligible population in each state should have become participants in the EPSDT program. Some states have a long way to go.

In the past, states had broad discretion in deciding which EPSDT services would be provided to which populations of Medicaid-eligible children. This discretion no longer exists. Key language in the present legislation requires necessary treatment services to correct or ameliorate a defect, physical or mental illness, or condition discovered during the screening examination. If a health care procedure is required—diagnostic, treatment, or follow-up service—it must be provided as an EPSDT service even if these services are not contained in the state Medicaid plan. OBRA-1989 can potentially increase access to services because there is greater federal financial intervention in provider rate-setting. Eligibility expansions for Medicaid are limited to prenatal care for the unborn child and primary and preventive services for children under six years of age with family incomes below 133% of the poverty line. However, making more children eligible for Medicaid will not solve the problems in child health or in the functioning of the EPSDT program. The eligibility expansions will automatically increase the number of eligibles, and the problems that are inherent in the system will be exacerbated. For example, since most states are reaching only a small percentage of their eligible population, the problems that affect state enrollment and participation may worsen as the number of eligible children increases.

HOW MANY CHILDREN ARE BEING REACHED BY EPSDT?

According to Hill and Breyel (1991), the American Academy of Pediatrics found that in 1989, only 22% of the Medicaid-eligible children received EPSDT services, and on average, 1.3% of state Medicaid budgets were spent on EPSDT. Although Medicaid is the major source of funding for child health services, only a quarter of the Medicaid expenditures are spent on basic health services for children. At least three-quarters of all Medicaid expenditures are spent on services for the aged, blind, and disabled adults (Sardell, 1990). In the state of Pennsylvania approximately 1% to 1.5% of the state's $2.2 billion Medicaid budget is spent on EPSDT services (Carr, 1989; Hanks, 1989). Since so few children are receiving basic preventive services through Medicaid's EPSDT program, and because the program has been around for more than 20 years, restructuring may be needed so that more eligible children can be reached.

Over the last six years, data collected from EPSDT programs nationwide show increased EPSDT participation rates for some states and a constant or decreased participation rate for others (see Figure 8.1). The Annual EPSDT Performance Indicator reports for 1985 to 1990 provide information on the percentage of eligible children who participate in the program in each state. These reports by the Health Care Financing Administration (HCFA) are compiled yearly from the quarterly reports (HCFA-420) of each state EPSDT program.[2] One of the limitations of the federal data is that it is very difficult to confirm children's participation in EPSDT across states because of the varying interpretations of the federal reporting guidelines by state officials (Hill and Breyel, 1991). However, the data collected by HCFA are the only source of nationwide information we have with which to examine the extent to which EPSDT is reaching its eligible population nationwide.

The annual participation rate for EPSDT programs in 1990 was approximately 38.9% of the eligible population. The participation ratio ranged from a high of 90% of the eligible population in one state to a low of less than 10% of the eligible population in others (see Figure 8.1). In 1990, 33 state programs had less than 50% of their eligible population enrolled in the EPSDT program, while 17 programs had 50% or more enrolled. For the last six years, some state programs have consistently failed to reach acceptable numbers of their eligible population.

Six of the 17 programs that reached 50% or more of their eligible population in 1990 are in the same region—Region III—which includes Tennessee (50.5%), Alabama (56.1%), Florida (69%), Mississippi (57.6%), North Carolina (60.5%), and South Carolina (90.6%). Of the ten regions listed, Region III has the best record for reaching high percentages of their eligible population (Figure 8.2). Three of the programs in Region III—Georgia, South Carolina, and Tennessee—contract with the Office of Maternal and Child Health services programs to administer their EPSDT programs while the remaining states—Alabama, Florida, Kentucky, Mississippi, and North Carolina—administer their programs through welfare eligibility offices.

FIGURE 8.1. State EPSDT Programs FY* 1985–1990 Participation Ratios

STATE	FY 1985	FY 1986	FY 1987	FY 1988	FY 1989	FY 1990
South Carolina	42.7	55.5	61.8	68.5	78.9	90.6
Wyoming	26.3	22.8	17.7	21.3	26.8	75.3
Colorado	54.1	41.3	30.7	89.9	68.4	70.8
Alaska	51.8	52.9	54.2	41.8	49.1	70.6
Florida	43.0	48.9	50.8	50.7	59.1	69.0
Vermont	56.2	42.6	58.0	60.1	67.7	67.1
Utah	35.8	20.5	15.6	20.4	39.9	64.0
North Carolina	37.7	49.9	50.1	45.6	53.9	60.5
Virginia	65.5	63.0	61.6	61.8	52.1	60.2
West Virginia	43.0	50.3	52.9	48.7	56.0	59.4
California	42.6	45.6	48.7	49.3	49.8	58.1
Mississippi	30.7	28.5	31.3	27.6	32.9	57.6
Nebraska	60.3	48.6	45.5	50.0	57.1	56.7
Alabama	12.5	20.4	29.7	40.4	40.1	56.1
Montana	13.6	35.1	27.7	34.1	41.7	54.1
Arkansas	12.6	8.3	6.3	7.9	27.5	52.8
Tennessee	29.3	43.9	26.6	24.0	24.3	50.5
Georgia	20.6	33.9	36.2	46.7	44.0	49.2
Nevada	44.9	51.7	48.0	47.0	49.2	47.8
Massachusetts	42.1	47.6	45.4	45.1	51.6	47.6
Rhode Island	46.4	47.8	28.8	40.7	44.3	45.2
Maine	16.8	17.0	45.5	51.1	55.0	45.1
Illinois	29.8	33.9	30.0	35.6	46.2	43.9
Louisiana	12.6	19.9	32.0	32.9	33.1	42.6
Hawaii	10.1	7.2	21.0	26.3	27.8	40.9
Maryland	21.5	32.1	25.5	25.9	31.7	32.8
Pennsylvania	23.8	24.2	23.7	28.5	31.4	32.6
Missouri	16.9	21.4	21.3	19.2	24.2	32.2
Ohio	25.1	48.2	32.9	30.6	34.6	31.9
Oregon	23.1	24.5	21.5	15.7	10.1	29.9
Arizona	6.2	13.8	17.7	31.0	35.7	29.8
New Mexico	16.6	17.3	18.6	24.1	35.2	29.7
Washington	15.5	13.1	15.0	28.9	29.2	27.5
Minnesota	23.0	21.2	20.4	21.2	23.1	26.0
South Dakota	18.1	14.7	16.4	16.2	21.0	25.2
Texas	25.2	25.6	21.8	22.0	23.5	25.2
North Dakota	25.8	24.8	23.0	18.1	18.8	24.0

* Fiscal Year

FIGURE 8.1 (continued)

STATE	FY 1985	FY 1986	FY 1987	FY 1988	FY 1989	FY 1990
District of Columbia	17.5	31.4	23.6	27.3	24.3	20.2
Michigan	19.2	19.2	20.8	20.0	20.7	19.9
Connecticut	15.5	13.8	13.3	15.8	9.7	14.0
Idaho	17.2	16.6	15.9	15.6	11.6	13.3
Kentucky	9.0	10.0	9.5	8.4	13.3	13.2
Kansas	11.5	7.4	31.4	21.9	12.8	13.0
New York	11.9	15.0	13.6	12.8	12.8	12.4
Oklahoma	14.4	6.6	21.4	15.7	7.0	10.4
New Jersey	11.0	11.1	10.2	10.4	9.5	9.6
Delaware	10.8	10.2	8.7	8.1	6.9	9.4
Wisconsin	10.8	8.8	7.7	7.4	9.5	9.4
Indiana	7.8	9.0	7.3	9.0	8.7	9.1
New Hampshire	15.0	10.2	12.5	12.1	10.9	9.1

In addition to the low enrollment of participants, the number of physicians that are willing to participate in Medicaid has decreased. The changes in OBRA-1989 increases the number of eligibles and the amount of reimbursements to encourage provider participation, but higher reimbursements and larger pools of eligibles are not the only factors physicians consider when providing care to the poor.

LOW PROVIDER PARTICIPATION: A BARRIER TO ACCESS

In an effort to contain cost, regulatory changes over the years have made the Medicaid program very rigid and complex (Perloff, Kletke, and Neckerman, 1987). The threat to professional autonomy posed by cost control strategies provides few incentives for provider participation. Providers are categorized by (1) those who participate and (2) those who participate on a limited basis in the Medicaid program (National Center for Children in Poverty, 1990; American Academy of Pediatrics, 1990). Between 1978 and 1989, the number of pediatricians treating any Medicaid recipients declined from 85% to 77%, while those with limited participation, who see only some of the recipients who request care, increased

FIGURE 8.2. State EPSDT Programs in FY 1985–1990 Participation Ratios by Region

STATE	FY 1985	FY 1986	FY 1987	FY 1988	FY 1989	FY 1990
Connecticut	15.5	13.8	13.3	15.8	9.7	14.0
Maine	16.8	17.0	45.5	51.1	55.0	45.1
Massachusetts	42.1	47.6	45.4	45.1	51.6	47.6
New Hampshire	15.0	10.2	12.5	12.1	10.9	9.1
Rhode Island	46.4	47.8	28.8	40.7	44.3	45.2
Vermont	56.2	42.6	58.0	60.1	67.7	67.1
Total Region I						
New Jersey	11.0	11.1	10.2	10.4	9.5	9.6
New York	11.9	15.0	13.6	12.8	12.8	12.4
Total Region II						
Delaware	10.8	10.2	8.7	8.1	6.9	9.4
District of Columbia	17.5	31.4	23.6	27.3	24.3	20.2
Maryland	21.5	32.1	25.5	25.9	31.7	32.8
Pennsylvania	23.8	24.2	23.7	28.5	31.4	32.6
Virginia	65.5	63.0	61.6	61.8	52.1	60.2
West Virginia	43.0	50.3	52.9	48.7	56.0	59.4
Total Region III						
Alabama	12.5	20.4	29.7	40.4	40.1	56.1
Florida	43.0	48.9	50.8	50.7	59.1	69.0
Georgia	20.6	33.9	36.2	46.7	44.0	49.2
Kentucky	9.0	10.0	9.5	8.4	13.3	13.2
Mississippi	30.7	28.5	31.3	27.6	32.9	57.6
North Carolina	37.7	49.9	50.1	45.6	53.9	60.5
South Carolina	42.7	55.5	61.8	68.5	78.9	90.6
Tennessee	29.3	43.9	26.6	24.0	24.3	50.5
Total Region IV						
Illinois	29.8	33.9	30.0	35.6	46.2	43.9
Indiana	7.8	9.0	7.3	9.0	8.7	9.1

FIGURE 8.2 (continued)

STATE	FY 1985	FY 1986	FY 1987	FY 1988	FY 1989	FY 1990
Michigan	19.2	19.2	20.8	20.0	20.7	19.9
Minnesota	23.0	21.2	20.4	21.2	23.1	26.0
Ohio	25.1	48.2	32.9	30.6	34.6	31.9
Wisconsin	10.8	8.8	7.7	7.4	9.5	9.4
Total Region V						
Arkansas	12.6	8.3	6.3	7.9	27.5	52.8
Louisiana	12.6	19.9	32.0	32.9	33.1	42.6
New Mexico	16.6	17.3	18.6	24.1	35.2	29.7
Oklahoma	14.4	6.6	21.4	15.7	7.0	10.4
Texas	25.2	25.6	21.8	22.0	23.5	25.2
Total Region VI						
Iowa	14.6	11.7	10.7	9.6	8.8	8.4
Kansas	11.5	7.4	31.4	21.9	12.8	13.0
Missouri	16.9	21.4	21.3	19.2	24.2	32.2
Nebraska	60.3	48.6	45.5	50.0	57.1	56.7
Total Region VII						
Colorado	54.1	41.3	30.7	89.9	68.4	70.8
Montana	13.6	35.1	27.7	34.1	41.7	54.1
North Dakota	25.8	24.8	23.0	18.1	18.8	24.0
South Dakota	18.8	14.7	16.4	16.2	21.0	25.2
Utah	35.8	20.5	15.6	20.4	39.9	64.0
Wyoming	26.3	22.8	17.7	21.3	26.8	75.3
Total Region VIII						
Arizona	6.2	13.8	17.7	31.0	35.7	29.8
California	42.6	45.6	48.7	49.3	49.8	58.1
Hawaii	10.1	7.2	21.0	26.3	27.8	40.9
Nevada	44.9	51.7	48.0	47.0	49.2	47.8
Total Region IX						
Alaska	51.8	52.9	54.2	41.8	49.1	70.6
Idaho	17.2	16.6	15.9	15.6	11.6	13.3
Oregon	23.1	24.5	21.5	15.7	10.1	29.9
Washington	15.5	13.1	15.0	28.9	29.2	27.5
Total Region X						

from 26% to 39%. Low reimbursement fee levels and administrative red tape are consistently given as reasons for low participation in Medicaid programs (Mitchell, 1991; Holleman et al., 1991).

In addition, Medicaid and Pediatric Primary Care (Perloff, Kletke, and Neckerman, 1987), a report supported by the American Academy of Pediatrics and funded by Health Care Financing Administration (HCFA), contended that when physicians provide services to Medicaid recipients they lose control and autonomy because federal regulations place restrictions on what procedures physicians can and cannot perform if they want to be reimbursed for their services. Furthermore, insurance companies and other payers assert that doctors often provide unnecessary costly services that are not always warranted; therefore cost controls are needed.

In a comparison of participation rates for two comparable groups of physicians in 1977 to 1978 and 1984 to 1985, Mitchell (1991) found a small but statistically significant decline in the overall participation rates for physicians, from 12.1% in 1977 to 1978 to 9.5% in 1984 to 1985. While the percentage of physicians accepting at least some Medicaid patients has increased from 77.3% to 83.5%, the average participation rate of all physicians has decreased. However, within the subspeciality areas of pediatrics and obstetrics/gynecology, both the percentage of providers and the average participation rates have increased. Mitchell further states that physicians in rural areas are more likely to accept Medicaid patients and have a larger Medicaid practice when compared to urban physicians.

The OBRA-1989 provisions require an increase in Medicaid fees, relative to what private payers will pay, and expansions in recipient eligibility to increase the demand for Medicaid services to encourage more provider participation. However, when state officials impose limits on the quantity of services and require prior authorizations before some services can be provided, this federal incentive is nullified. The quantity of services permissible and the need for prior authorizations will restrict the supply of physician visits and create additional red tape (Mitchell, 1991).

But marginal fees are not the only reason providers do not participate in Medicaid. In a study of "Uncompensated Outpatient Medical Care by Physicians" (Holleman et al., 1991), physicians listed the following problems in providing care to the poor: (1) the inappropriate use of medical care by the medically indigent, (2) lack of government financial support, (3) high cost of health care, and (4) legal liability. Physicians believe that the poor wait until their problems are severe before seeing physicians and they are less likely to return for follow-up care. They believe the lack of government funding, at both the federal and state levels, is responsible for the crisis in medical care for the poor. The duplication of government programs, without central access, and the limitations of Medicare and Medicaid create difficulties (Holleman et al., 1991). Every program has separate eligibility requirements and service restrictions. With the exception of Medicare, which is a universal program, publicly funded medical programs for the poor are decentralized between state and local governments. Although some physicians provide the initial evaluations for those unable to pay, the laboratory, radiology, medication, and follow-up costs make complete evaluations very difficult. When financial barriers make total care (e.g., diagnostic testing, referrals, and hospitalization) impossible, there is a belief that treating poor patients at risk increases the likelihood of malpractice suits (Holleman et al., 1991).

In addition to the above, some providers have negative stereotypes about the race and status of Medicaid recipients and are unwilling to have poor people in their waiting rooms (National Center for Clinical Infant Programs, 1990; Institute of Medicine, 1988). According to the Institute of Medicine (1988), traditional medical care is overburdened by middle-class value systems that have failed to provide essential services to significant sectors of the population. The system needs to be more sensitive to values of women, minorities, and other neglected groups. The stigma that is attached to Medicaid as a welfare program also impacts provider participation in the EPSDT program. Providers view EPSDT as a welfare program because they are reimbursed through state Medicaid budgets.

If EPSDT is located within state departments of health nationwide, public health personnel—physicans, nurses, and others—could help meet the demand for health services through MCH services programs, crippled children's programs, well-child care and baby clinics, and local community health centers. A combined comprehensive program could centralize access to child health services within

the states, decrease duplication, consolidate eligibility requirements, and ease service restrictions.

HOW SHOULD EPSDT BE ADMINISTERED?

A major problem with EPSDT lies within the way it is administered. The decision regarding where to place administrative responsibility for EPSDT has been crucial to its effectiveness. Ironically,
the issue goes back to 1967 when Congress was debating EPSDT as
a health or a welfare program. The program was administratively
placed in the welfare bureaucracy, but over the years legislative
changes at the federal level have strengthened it as a child health
program. Where a program is structurally placed in the bureaucracy
determines how it will be administered (Copeland, 1992a; Van
Horn and Van Meter, 1975). According to Hill and Breyel (1991),
"administrative design decisions influence how the program inter-
acts with its recipients" (p. 39). The way in which program officials
coordinate service delivery for the EPSDT program (e.g., help families locate providers, make appointments, remember periodic
screens, and arrange transportation) is crucial for many states.

Most EPSDT programs are administered in one of two ways. In
28 states, administration of the EPSDT program is the responsibility of the Medicaid-eligibility agency located in public welfare
offices. In 16 states, administrative responsibility for the EPSDT
program is under the jurisdiction of the Maternal and Child Health
services program located in the local health department. Two states
use community agencies that include MCH services, and one state
uses a private nonprofit organization to administer EPSDT.

One of the questions that is repeatedly asked about the EPSDT
programs is whether there is a difference between EPSDT programs
that are administered by state welfare offices and those administered by state health offices. There are clearly some structural as
well as philosophical differences in the health versus welfare
bureaucracies. The training of officials, and as well, the primary
mission of each agency, are different. Title XIX operates as an
insurance reimbursement system for poor families, whereas Title V
operates as a public health care delivery system. In addition, Title V
services are publicly funded projects that assume an obligation to

service specifically defined populations—women and children. Nine of the 17 states that are reaching 50% or more of their eligible populations are subcontracting their EPSDT program to Maternal and Child Health services programs.

Many of the states using the welfare eligibility-based EPSDT administration are dissatisfied with this approach (Hill and Breyel, 1991). Connecting EPSDT to the public assistance eligibility process undermines the effectiveness of the program. The traditional role of public assistance in the United States gives recipients a feeling of being stigmatized (Bullough and Bullough, 1982; Karger and Stoesz, 1990; Klerman, 1991). The nature of welfare is so demeaning that recipients feel uncomfortable and embarrassed asking for assistance. According to Klerman (1991), at times people will do without health benefits rather than seek help at a welfare office. Public health services do not have this negative association, as they are part of the mainstream public services. Due to the demeaning nature of welfare assistance, as well as the sometimes hostile environment that surrounds it, it is not surprising that some people are more willing to ask for health care services that are not stamped with the negative welfare label (Institute of Medicine, 1988).

In addition, the National Governors Association found that states administering their EPSDT program through MCH or other agencies generally believe their programs are more successful. They reach a higher percentage of eligibles, they are administered as health service delivery programs, health professionals assume the case manager role and are more effective in communicating the value of health care services, and the emphasis is on the quality of services rather than cost control. Program managers, clients, and MCH and Medicaid officials believe that EPSDT has a stronger identity as a health care program when administration is conducted by agencies other than welfare departments. In most of these states where the person who is contacting the family is a public health provider, EPSDT as an important health care benefit is communicated more convincingly. Delinking EPSDT management from the eligibility process reduces client confusion; clarifies roles and responsibilities among public program staff; and, instead of forcing eligibility specialists to also manage a preventive health program, state officials can rely on health care providers to do the job they are best equipped to do (Hill and Breyel, 1991). Of the states surveyed, 32 believe that connection through the eligibility system is negative and only nine believe it is positive.

IMPROVING EPSDT

EPSDT has helped to improve the health status of poor children while decreasing the cost of their medical care. Sardell (1990) notes that "[c]hildren with Medicaid have higher utilization rates of medical care than do low-income children without public health insurance" (p. 278). A study evaluating the EPSDT program in the state of Michigan revealed that medical costs for children participating in EPSDT were nearly 13% lower than those for nonparticipating eligible children (Klerman, 1991). The Michigan study showed that children who received frequent periodic screens needed fewer referrals for medical problems. A Pennsylvania study showed that children with health problems at the time of the initial EPSDT screening had the problem resolved by the time of the rescreening, and that participating eligibles had lower rates of hospital admissions and physician visits. Studies from Ohio, North Dakota, Virginia, and North Carolina also showed that EPSDT participation improved health status and reduced medical cost (Hill and Breyel, 1991; Klerman, 1991). However, the program's low participation rates nationwide indicate that it is failing to achieve its full potential.

For EPSDT to reach its full potential, state officials need to consider integrating it into the broader health care program and thereby building one comprehensive health care program to meet the needs of all poor children. There are positive features of both the EPSDT and MCH services programs that could be combined. Separately, the programs offer some unique services, but they also overlap and duplicate services. The target populations of both programs are low-income families with children. The welfare bureaucracy needs to be convinced of the value of EPSDT and the problems of administering a child health service delivery program in a health reimbursement system. The welfare bureaucracy, in most states, is not as appropriate as the health bureaucracy to develop, design, implement, administer, and monitor the content and quality of health services (Copeland, 1992a; Klerman, 1991; Children's

Defense Fund, 1977). The preliminary data suggest that in the majority of states with collaborating agreements between Title XIX and Title V programs, EPSDT is more effective, and that as a comprehensive health care program for children, EPSDT is more effective in a health bureaucracy than a welfare bureaucracy. Title V has a long history of developing and providing comprehensive primary and preventive health services to low-income women and children. A well-coordinated comprehensive child health system under one agency may be much more efficient in handling the health care needs of poor children.

As an incremental approach to the crisis in the health care system, and as a long-term strategy for children, this is likely to be a more cost-effective way to provide child health services with universal access while preventing the expensive overlap and duplication of services provided by two separate programs. If EPSDT and MCH were combined, EPSDT could be the entry point for continuing care through the MCH programs. Then, the MCH services program could be the centralized accessing organization for comprehensive child health services for all poor and low-income children. If restructured appropriately, such a program would alleviate the fragmentation in the present child health service delivery system.

To restructure the system to meet the needs of more children, state officials would have to assess the present operations of their EPSDT programs to examine their participation ratios and whether their programs are effectively linked with other service delivery systems for children. If the state annual participation ratios are consistently low and if EPSDT is not integrated with other child health programs, restructuring is most appropriate. If restructuring seems unlikely, progress is possible only through greater collaboration between Title XIX and Title V administrators at both the national and state levels.

CONCLUSION

The immediate adoption of a national health program that combines all child health services, from Title XIX and Title V, would provide equitable access to all medical and health services. Such a program would help to alleviate the existing financial, systemic, and knowledge barriers to health care for poor children. Limited access to health care services for some will not meet the need for a universal access program for all. But until we can develop a health care system that is available and affordable to everyone, some groups will gain while other groups will lose. This is only an incremental approach, and not the best solution to our present health crisis. However, improving child health services is a major priority, and at this time combining these two programs may be more feasible than broad-based reform. An integration of the two major child health programs may be a politically practical and efficient way to provide all children with access to more effective health services at or close to the same levels of funding.

NOTES

1. "As a comprehensive child health program . . . EPSDT consists of two mutually supportive, operational components: assuring the availability and accessibility of required health resources and helping Medicaid recipients and their parents or guardians effectively use them. These components enable Medicaid agencies to manage a comprehensive child health program of prevention and treatment, to systematically: (1) seek out eligibles and inform them of the benefits of prevention and the health services and assistance available; (2) help them and their families use health resources, including their own talents and knowledge, effectively and efficiently; (3) assess the child's health needs through initial and periodic examinations and evaluation; and (4) assure that health problems found are diagnosed and treated early, before they become more complex and their treatment more costly" (DHHS, 1988, Transmittal #2, Section 5, p. 3).

2. The HCFA-420 reports submitted by EPSDT program officials list: (1) the number of children eligible for EPSDT; (2) the number enrolled in continuing care arrangements; (3) the number receiving screening services; (4) the total number of screens performed; and (5) the number of eligibles referred for corrective treatment. By adding the number of children in continuing care to the number of children that have received screens and dividing this sum by the total number of eligibles, a participation ratio is calculated. Similarly, if the total number of screens performed is divided by the total number of eligibles, a screening ratio is derived (Hill and Breyel, 1991).

REFERENCES

American Academy of Pediatrics (AAP) (1989). AAP Special Report. *Barriers to Care.* Grove Village: AAP.

American Academy of Pediatrics (1990). AAP Special Report. *Solutions.* Grove Village: AAP.

Bergman, A.I. (1990). "In-Depth Review of OBRA." Paper presented at *Making Change Happen: Fifth Annual Maternal & Child Health Leadership Conference.* Chicago: March 28, 1990.

Bullough, V.L., and Bullough, B. (1982). *Health Care for the Other Americans.* New York: Appleton-Century-Crofts.

Carr, V.R. (1989). *The Implementation Process as a Framework for Policy Analysis.* Doctoral Dissertation, University of Pittsburgh.

Children's Defense Fund (1977). *EPSDT: Does it Spell Health Care for Poor Children?* Washington, DC: Washington Research Project, Inc.

Copeland, V.C. (1992a). "The Policy Implementation Process as a Framework for Policy Analysis." Paper presented at the *Council on Social Work Annual Program Meeting.* Kansas: March 3, 1992.

Copeland, V.C. (1992b). "What Happened to EPSDT in the State of Pennsylvania." Unpublished Manuscript.

Department of Health and Human Services (DHHS). (1981). *The Select Panel for the Promotion of Child Health: Better Health for Our Children: A National Strategy.* Pub. No. (PHS) 7955071.

Department of Health and Human Services (DHHS). (1988). *State Medicaid Manual Part 5—Early and Periodic Screening, Diagnosis, and Treatment (EPSDT).* Transmittal #2. Washington, DC: Health Care Financing Administration.

Department of Health and Human Services (DHHS). (1990). *Prevention '89/'90: Federal Programs and Progress.* U.S. Government Printing Office: Washington, DC.

Foltz, A.M. (1975). "The Development of Ambiguous Federal Policy: Early and Periodic Screening Diagnosis and Treatment." *Millbank Memorial Quarterly* 53, Winter, 35–63.

Hanks, F. (February, 1989). Personal Interview.

Hanlon, J.J., and Pickett, G. (1984). *Public Health Administration and Practice.* Santa Clara: Times Mirror.

Hill, I.T., and Breyel, J.M. (1991). *Caring for Kids.* Washington, DC: National Governors' Association.

Holleman, M.C., Loe, H.D., Selwyn, B.J., and Kapadia, A. (1991). "Uncompensated Outpatient Medical Care by Physicians." *Medical Care,* Vol. 29, No. 7, July.

Institute of Medicine (1988). *The Future of Public Health.* The Committee for the Study of the Future of Public Health Services. Division of Health Services, Institute of Medicine. Washington, DC: National Academy Press.

Karger, H.J., and Stoesz, D. (1990). *American Social Welfare Policy: A Structural Approach.* White Plains: Longman.

Klerman, L.V. (1991). *Alive and Well.* New York: Columbia University.

Mitchell, J.B. (1991). "Physician Participation in Medicaid." *Medical Care,* Vol. 29, No. 7, July.

National Center for Children in Poverty. (1990). *Five Million Children.* New York: Columbia University.

National Center for Clinical Infant Programs. (1990). *February Update: Medicaid Expansions.* Washington, DC: Dave Chavkin.

National Commission on Children (NCC). (1991). *Beyond Rhetoric—A New American Agenda for Children and Families: Final Report of The National Commission on Children.* Washington, DC: U.S. Government Printing Office.

National Commission to Prevent Infant Mortality. (1990). *Troubling Trends: The Health of America's Next Generation.* Washington: National Commission to Prevent Infant Mortality.

Perloff, J.D., Kletke, P.R., and Neckerman, K.M. (1987). *Medicaid and Pediatric Primary Care.* Baltimore: Johns Hopkins Press.

Sardell, A. (1990). "Child Health Policy in the U.S.: The Paradox of Consensus." *Journal of Health Politics, Policy, and Law,* Vol. 15, #2, Summer.

Van Horn, C.E., and Van Meter, D.S. (1975). "The Policy Implementation Process: A Conceptual Framework." *Administration and Society,* February, Vol. 6, #4, pp. 445–488.

Chapter 9

Interventions and Policies to Serve Homeless People Infected with HIV and AIDS

Madeleine R. Stoner

INTRODUCTION

Acquired immune deficiency syndrome (AIDS) epidemiologic investigations conducted by the Centers for Disease Control (CDC) indicate widespread human immunodeficiency virus (HIV) seroprevalence rates among homeless people. These rates are disproportionately higher among homeless people than the domiciled population. CDC data, along with other recent studies, confirm anecdotal information and experiences emanating from homeless advocates and service providers who allege that HIV, AIDS, and other communicable diseases are increasing within homeless populations. This convergence of two of the most serious problems of our day is beginning to be addressed at program and policy levels, but much remains to be done.

The spread of HIV and AIDS among homeless people demands greater attention from social workers and all health service professionals so that education, prevention, and treatment can follow. In addition to the more humane concerns about social pathology, public health concerns pose a strong imperative for action. Shelter staff, and other homeless service providers, must develop new skills to

---

This chapter was previously published in *Journal of Health & Social Policy*, Vol. 7(1) 1995.

adequately respond to the needs of HIV-infected homeless people, as well as those who have not contracted the infection but are highly susceptible. These perspectives demand equal attention from human service providers to protect homeless people who are infected, those who are not infected, as well as the domiciled population.

This chapter presents surveillance data on the scope of HIV seroprevalence and AIDS among homeless people. It describes sequences of behavior and events that lead homeless people to become infected and recommends intervention strategies and policies that address the unmet needs of HIV/AIDS-infected homeless people. It notes that barriers to care that exist for all indigent people are exacerbated by stigma, organizational domain conflicts, and too few specialized facilities for homeless infected people.

Acknowledging that federal funding for HIV and AIDS has addressed some of the need for medical care, supportive services, and housing, preliminary assessment of these programs is offered. Finally, the chapter presents data demonstrating that homeless people do respond to incentives for behavioral change and safe acts. These data justify the development of broad based AIDS education and prevention interventions on the part of homeless service providers and health care practitioners.

EPIDEMIOLOGICAL DATA

The CDC reported that the AIDS virus has infected the nation's homeless at rates that are two to 40 times as high as those of the domiciled population. Medical data, collected for 8,000 homeless people in 13 cities, indicate that 1% to 20% of the subjects are infected with the HIV infection, depending upon the cities surveyed. Nationally, the rate of infection is estimated to be less than 0.5%.[1]

Luna (1990) found that the HIV infection is currently spreading most rapidly among the nation's disenfranchised and those least likely to protect themselves. This pattern is evident among several cohorts of homeless people, most notably adolescents who are at extremely high risk of HIV infection. The seropositivity rate for this population is two to ten times higher than the rate reported for other adolescent samples in the United States.[2] Stricof et al. found HIV seroprevalence among 4% of homeless adolescents.[3]

Three subgroups of adolescents in the general population are most at risk of HIV seroprevalence: (1) gay and lesbian adolescents; (2) sexually abused youth; and, (3) drug abusers. Six percent of homeless adolescents identify themselves as gay or lesbian.[4] Sixty percent of homeless youth report having been sexually active.[5] Thirty-nine percent of homeless youth have sold drugs to support their habits, or for income.[6] Twenty-eight percent use crack-cocaine, which is closely associated with HIV seropositivity.[7]

Sexual risk behaviors are more common among homeless youth than among those who are domiciled. Although similar percentages of homeless and nonhomeless young people engage in sexual activity, homeless youth have more sex partners and become sexually active approximately two years earlier than their housed counterparts.[8]

These data clearly reveal the high risk status of homeless youth. They derive their risk not only from sexual and substance abuse behaviors, but also from their concentrations in neighborhoods with high HIV seroprevalence rates.

In the adult homeless population, the fastest growing rate of infection is occurring among crack-cocaine users. This is particularly so in cities like New York where large drug centers prevail within the drug culture.[9] However, the greatest number of homeless infected adults are gay and bisexual men.[10]

Scant attention has been paid to homeless infected women. Even the expanded CDC case definition of AIDS does not address the fact that HIV infection manifests itself differently in women than in men. No conclusive epidemiological data have been presented on HIV/AIDS prevalence among homeless women. CDC recorded rates for domiciled women are also unreliable. This is because physicians frequently overlook routine gynecological conditions such as genital herpes, yeast infections, and pelvic inflammatory disease as symptoms of HIV infection. The concentration on homosexual and bisexual males, and IV drug users, has condoned the definition of AIDS in terms of male symptoms so that women with HIV infection are being passed over.

Minority group women have the highest prevalence rates for HIV seroprevalence. They also comprise the largest cohort of homeless women. Overlap must exist between the two. African-American women and Latinas have been most affected by HIV infection. Seventy-four percent of women with AIDS, recorded by the CDC, are African-American. Intravenous drug use and sexual contact are the modes of transmission to these women.[11]

Homeless women generally receive no routine gynecological care. Many turn to prostitution for survival. Many are teenagers. Standard AIDS education and prevention is notably irrelevant for women who need food and must deal with the exigencies of homelessness.

Because African-American men comprise a disproportionate number of the homeless, it is clear that they will increasingly be infected with AIDS. The ethnic breakdown of patients who visit the Weingart Center located in Los Angeles' Skid Row, is approximately 60% African-American. National data indicate that 78% of all single homeless adults are men, mostly African American.[12]

The connection between tuberculosis and HIV infection poses particular problems for homeless people. Those infected with the HIV virus are highly susceptible to opportunistic infections, in particular, tuberculosis. A contagious disease associated with poverty, tuberculosis has spread rapidly. New York State, with the highest incidence of tuberculosis in the United States, has experienced more than a doubling in the number of active tuberculosis cases since 1978. Eighty-four percent of these cases occur in New York City. Homeless people have been more exposed to tuberculosis than domiciled people, and are manifesting a higher rate of tuberculosis. The Centers for Disease Control estimates the tuberculosis rate to be from 1.6% to 6.8% among homeless people living in shelters. This rate is 150 times higher than that of the general population.[13]

This problem is further complicated by two situations. It is extremely difficult to diagnose tuberculosis among people who are co-infected with HIV; and new strains of tuberculosis are proving to be resistant to drugs.[14]

PATTERNS OF HIV/AIDS HOMELESS POPULATIONS

Brickner et al.[15] and more recently, the Committee on Health Care for Homeless People organized by the National Academy of Science Institute of Medicine, noted that homeless people are at relatively high risk for a wide range of acute and chronic illnesses. In examining the relationship between homelessness and illness,

Brickner et al. identified three discrete interactions. Some health problems precede and contribute to homelessness. Others are a consequence of homelessness. The third occurs when the condition of homelessness complicates treatment.[16] One typology of analyzing HIV-infected homeless people is to view them as two separate populations according to whether HIV or homelessness occurred first.[17]

The first sequence refers to situations in which the progress of a disease leads to repeated and more serious bouts with opportunistic infections forcing infected individuals out of work, and ultimately, unable to pay rent. AIDS is a primary example of an illness that leads to homelessness because of resource exhaustion. The following case study illustrates this cycle:

> A divorced Anglo-African woman, in her mid-thirties, left her family in England to pursue an entrepreneurial venture in the cosmetics industry. She arrived in Los Angeles and proceeded to search for capital to develop her business. After unsuccessful medical treatment for eczema, she was diagnosed as HIV positive with a T-cell count of 500. Within six months she exhausted her venture capital, could no longer pay her rent and ended at the Weingart Center on Los Angeles' Skid Row.

The second set of identified connections between homelessness and illness in which homelessness leads to disease, is prominently displayed among homeless adolescents and youth.

> A nineteen-year-old male college student exhausted all funds and personal resources as a result of his addiction to crack-cocaine. Forced to live in the street, his habit became a trigger for unsafe acts. Despite his large and healthy appearance, he was diagnosed as HIV positive with a CD4 count of < 200.

Because substance abuse, sexually transmitted diseases, and pregnancy are more prevalent among homeless youth and adolescents than those in the domiciled population, HIV seroprevalence has emerged as an outcome of homeless life.[18]

The third sequence occurs when patterns of behavior and unhealthy conditions associated with homelessness complicate treatment. Crowded living in homeless shelters inhibits tuberculosis and

HIV-infected patients from maintaining a noninfectious regimen. Indeed, crowded living in shelters or streets presents the most extreme conditions for opportunistic infections.

Shelter regulations frequently prevent HIV-infected residents from getting sufficient rest. "Night sweats," a frequent malady for HIV-infected people on medication, force sleeplessness. Shelter rules that require everyone to awaken early ignore the special sleep needs of these people. The last step in this sequence of events occurs when the infected person decides not to take his or her medication because it is too difficult to comply with a treatment regimen when homeless.

The purpose of explaining the different sequences of events and conditions that connect homelessness and HIV/AIDS infection is to corroborate the general observations of homeless service providers who have been advocating for increased attention to the problem. Reports that greater numbers of people with AIDS are requesting services, and that many are unable to obtain emergency shelter, are now supported by aggregate data. The untested assumptions that the condition of homelessness is inextricably linked to the HIV/AIDS virus, either as antecedent or result, demand attention.

SERVICE AND RESOURCE BARRIERS FOR HIV/AIDS-INFECTED HOMELESS PEOPLE

Political, agency, diagnostic, and personal life style realities combine to pose a series of obstacles to effective responses to homeless HIV/AIDS-infected people.

The multiple life stressors, situations, and psychological adjustment problems of homeless people complicate all extant education, prevention, and HIV/AIDS treatment programs. Limited housing alternatives, lack of family support, and distress associated with the perils of homelessness mitigate against motivation to seek and use services. Other aspects of homeless life styles—in particular, sexual promiscuity and substance abuse—are so chaotic that standard education and prevention strategies, including testing, are difficult to apply. Finally, the prevalence of many opportunistic infections in the streets and shelters threaten rapid deterioration of HIV/AIDS-infected people.

Stigma imposes a unique problem for homeless infected people. Either condition stigmatizes them. The presence of both in their lives produces dual stigma that frequently compels them to conceal the fact of their HIV seroprevalence.[19]

Service providers, like shelters and physicians, frequently turn away known HIV- and AIDS-infected people. Brickner et al. found that physicians frequently refuse to treat homeless people because they cannot deal with the homeless conditions that contribute to medical noncompliance. A more recent study of 400 of Southern California's 4,000 primary care physicians confirmed the long-held belief that many physicians remain inadequately informed about HIV and AIDS, and that one-third of all primary care physicians do not agree that they have a responsibility to treat persons with AIDS.[20]

This powerful combination of homeless life style conditions and stigma retards treatment for homeless HIV-infected people. The disease progresses more rapidly because homeless infected people tend to seek treatment only at advanced stages. The Homeless Outreach Program in Los Angeles reports that homeless people generally have between 18 and 24 months life expectancy between diagnosis and demise.[21]

The emergency shelter system has reacted to HIV and AIDS infection with confusion. Providers describe a legitimate dilemma. As shelter providers, their mission is to respond to the needs of all homeless people. This means that they have a responsibility to shelter people who are infected. They are equally responsible for protecting the health and safety of noninfected shelter residents and staff.

This dilemma is particularly acute in New York City which operates its shelter programs under a right to shelter upon demand.[22] New York has responded by allocating the former welfare hotels and Single Room Occupancy (SRO) hotels. Other cities like Boston, Seattle, and Los Angeles, not laboring under the right to shelter law, have begun to operate ambitious model programs for homeless persons with AIDS. All cities report extensive waiting lists for AIDS housing, except New York.

Federal laws prohibiting discrimination based upon disability confound shelter operators. They allege that homeless people with AIDS should not be lodged in shelters mainly to protect them from the many opportunistic infections prevalent there. Other shelter providers justify the exclusion of all HIV-infected clients because they are concerned that they will lose shelter volunteers who fear exposure to AIDS.

A preliminary finding by an administrative law judge for the New York City Commission on Human Rights determined that the Partnership for the Homeless, which operates 150 shelters, has discriminated since 1989 against homeless people who have the AIDS virus. The Partnership for the Homeless, the nation's largest network of private shelters, does operate one 12-bed residence for homeless people with AIDS and with related conditions. It has also advocated more housing for those infected by the virus. As an exemplary shelter provider, the Partnership's official accusation of discrimination reflects the dilemma faced by most shelter operators.

Politically, homeless advocacy organizations, and individuals focused on obtaining resources, legal sanctions, and public sympathy for homeless people, face an even more perplexing dilemma than shelter providers. Public advocacy and exposure of HIV and AIDS prevalence among homeless people could easily lead public officials and philanthropists to dismiss the homeless population as a group not worth any further allocation of resources because of the inevitability of death.

In addition to their concerns about potential backlash, advocates face a sense of collective helplessness. Confronted by minimal resources, public apathy, and stigma, even the most compassionate people can justifiably withhold support and services because they envision so little return on investing in homeless people who have a terminal condition. It seems fairer and more rational to target scarce resources to people who can be rehabilitated.

Divisions between providers over service domains pose organizational barriers that result in uncoordinated care. Although they share the same clients, homeless and AIDS providers function in separate service domains, with minimal collaboration. This means that a homeless person infected with HIV- and AIDS-related symptoms can be practically without care.

The current systems for HIV/AIDS and homelessness—shelters and inpatient or outpatient treatment facilities—are not designed to deal with the multiple problems homeless infected people present. The systems are designed either to deal with medical problems or general survival needs, but usually not both. Conflicts arise for service users of systems with different domains.

Typically, a homeless person with AIDS-related symptoms or HIV can receive medication at a clinic, return to a shelter, take the medication, and go to sleep. That person may have "night sweats" forcing sleeplessness. However, he or she will be unable to sleep-in the next morning because shelter rules frequently require everyone to be out of bed by 7:00 a.m. Scarce toilet facilities in shelters are particularly distressing for HIV/AIDS-infected people who experience frequent bouts of diarrhea. Eventually people abandon their medication regimens because they render homeless life even more difficult.

In Los Angeles County, collaboration between delivery systems at policy-making levels began in the early 1990s. The AIDS Homeless Task Force had no representation from the homeless network of providers, advocates, and clients until homeless activists protested the situation. This was also true until recently of the AIDS regional board, mandated to allocate AIDS funds to Los Angeles County under the Ryan White Comprehensive AIDS Resource Emergency (CARE) Act.

Service delivery programs are too frequently limited to treating either HIV/AIDS patients or homeless people. Few are equipped to do both. Among those that are, mentally ill homeless HIV-infected people pose yet another problem and are often refused housing and treatment.

Finally, the diagnostic definition of AIDS creates serious problems for all homeless people, especially women. The standard case definition, developed by the CDC in the early 1980s, was based upon male symptoms. Moreover, the case definition based upon a CD4 lymphocyte count above 200 has been irrelevant for all poor people who cannot afford general health care.

One objective for expanding the surveillance case definition to include HIV-infected persons with CD4 counts below 200 was to simplify the classification and reporting system. Another objective was consistent standards of medical care for all HIV-infected persons. Measures of CD4 lymphocytes are currently used to guide clinical and/or therapeutic actions for HIV-infected persons. Antiretroviral therapy was recommended for HIV-infected persons with a CD4 lymphocyte count < 500. Prophylaxis against pneumocystis carinii pneumonia is now recommended for all HIV-infected persons with CD4 lymphocyte counts < 200.[23]

Unfortunately, liberalized Social Security Administration regulations governing Supplemental Security Income benefits for HIV-infected people, the mainstay of people who are unable to support themselves, fail to include the revised standard definition of AIDS. This means that early detection of HIV-infected homeless youth, IV drug users, and women for purposes of diagnosis that determines disability allowances may not occur. Higher HIV disability criteria exist for women and IV drug users than for infected men and non-IV users.[24] A further complication lies in the fact that Supplemental Security Income benefits are not available to an individual who is HIV positive but still able-bodied.[25]

The maze of problems faced by homeless people (crises, stigma, unsafe acts, dangerous public health and sanitation, and inadequate access to general health care) coupled with limited public policies, conflicts over organizational domain, and diagnostic biases, impose dual discrimination against homeless people who are infected with HIV- or AIDS-related illnesses.

RECOMMENDED INTERVENTIONS

The most compelling recommendation calls for recognition of the extent of HIV/AIDS prevalence among homeless people, followed by medical care, housing, and supportive services. Homeless, infected people need the same health care and social support that domiciled and more affluent patients receive. This requires both categorical services and services that are integrated within present homeless agencies and health settings.

Categorical services designed specifically for the homeless environment would address the needs of homeless infected people as well as protect those who are not infected. These services include: (1) specialized treatment programs; (2) specialized shelter; and, (3) categorical funding to solve unique and persistent problems.

Establishment of a categorical service network for homeless HIV/AIDS-infected people poses a series of complex but manageable structural and ethical issues. Maintaining client confidentiality when agencies are allowed to share information essential to complete care is foremost. Staff in each agency must negotiate across boundaries with specificity and attention to explanations to clients stressing the content of informed consent. Most case management service models have developed precedents for such protection.

Categorical funding for homeless infected people would guarantee the care that has not yet been available. The homeless population has hardly received money or attention from major funding resources for HIV/AIDS. As an example, Los Angeles County received $7.8 million, excluding supplemental grants, under the Ryan White CARE Act for its first year of implementation. The total amount allocated for homeless people in that year was less than 2% of the county funds.[26] General county funding and other HIV/AIDS resources have followed this pattern so that no early intervention, outpatient, or inpatient facilities are located in the county's Skid Row area, despite the presence there of the second highest HIV seroprevalence rate in Los Angeles.[27]

In 1990, the United States Congress passed the National Affordable Housing Act, which includes Housing Opportunities for Persons with AIDS (HOPWA). This program created housing resources for those cities hardest hit by the HIV/AIDS epidemic, enabling them to fund a range of programs for people living with HIV disease, including AIDS housing information and coordination of services; short-term supported housing and services; rental-assistance; single-room-occupancy housing; and community residences and services. National funding for fiscal year 1993 was $100 million.[28]

No official data has been produced about the implementation of HOPWA because the programs are just completing the planning stage. However, current expenditure plans allocate only $200,000 out of $7.2 million for food and shelter for homeless persons.[29]

The situation in greater Los Angeles reflects a national crisis in public health. The majority of public health resources for HIV/AIDS have gone to communities that are neither poor, undereducated, nor underrepresented. All public health services have been strained by treating HIV/AIDS patients who would not normally be in the public system, leaving scant room for indigent people who have no other access to health care.[30] Homeless people have no access to care except that in the public sector, and they are largely excluded from these in the case of HIV/AIDS.

Categorical programs and facilities, such as shelters, hospices, and day treatment programs for homeless infected people, would address the fact that neither the AIDS nor the homeless service systems respond adequately to the combined needs of homeless people infected with the HIV/AIDS virus. Special needs facilities that combine food, shelter, and medical and psychological services are essential to redress this service imbalance.

Adequate health care can be provided only when housing needs are met.[31] Housing persons with HIV infection is extremely expensive. Prominent recommendations for this population feature a continuum of housing for persons with mild symptoms ranging to those at terminal stages. Ideally, housing should accommodate people at different stages of illness. An example of such housing exists in the life care communities available for older Americans.

Other special needs programs for homeless people offer the necessary guidelines for combining medical, psychological, and residential services. Transitional living facilities for homeless mentally ill people are a sound exemplar.[32] The prevalence of drug- and alcohol-free shelters and transitional living facilities provide another example of categorical programming for homeless people.

Within the homeless service network, all service providers need education and training sessions to improve their knowledge and skills about work with homeless HIV/AIDS clients. The Los Angeles Homeless Health Care Project has developed a curriculum to meet three goals relevant to the needs of providers: (1) to increase knowledge of issues of public benefits; (2) to improve shelter and case management services; and, (3) to improve communicable disease control measures among shelter staff and other agencies serving homeless people.

One reason for resistance to increasing resources for homeless HIV/AIDS-infected people lies in a general perception that behavior change is highly unlikely. This notion is refuted by data from three intensive prevention programs that demonstrate reductions in risk behaviors among homeless HIV-infected gay men and homeless youth.

Des Jarlais and Friedman (1991) identify social learning theory as the conceptual framework for each of these programs. They share the following elements: (1) a minimum of ten sessions; (2) assertiveness and coping skills training; (3) acquisition of knowledge and positive attitudes toward safe acts; (4) identification of individual personal risk behaviors; (5) structured and continuing support for behavior change; and, (6) group meetings to develop and enhance open support and social norms for safe acts.[33]

A program targeted toward homeless adolescents in shelters has featured an additional element. It utilizes a comprehensive care structure in which community agencies develop joint administrative protocols to anticipate crises and establish an active network of service providers.[34]

The link between HIV testing and successful reduction of risk acts was explored at a general medical clinic on Skid Row in Los Angeles. In July 1990, voluntary confidential HIV testing and counseling were offered to all clinic patients evaluated for syphilis. By April 1991, researchers obtained face-to-face information for 346 homeless people.

Overall, seroprevalence was 4%. HIV risk behaviors were reported by 69% of the sample. Eighty percent of the sample reported that they had changed their sexual behavior to reduce the risk of AIDS. Among IV drug users, 44% had stopped injecting; of those who continued to inject, 70% stopped sharing works; 12% shared works less frequently; and 24% began, or increased, sharing works.[35]

Data from these programs challenge stereotypes by demonstrating that homeless people are informed about HIV and some have responded to education and prevention interventions. These data offer sufficient encouragement for continuing efforts to increase and sustain behavior change in homeless people who are either infected or at high risk.

SUMMARY

This chapter has presented data identifying the high prevalence of HIV/AIDS among homeless people. It has illustrated different links between HIV seroprevalence and cohorts of homeless populations. Acknowledging that barriers to health care exist for all homeless people, the chapter has stressed that those infected with HIV/AIDS experience additional problems associated with stigma, lack of coordination between delivery systems, a paucity of categorical facilities, and limited diagnostic standards.

A central concern of this chapter has focused on the inequitable distribution of HIV/AIDS resources to homeless people. Even though the federal government has recently stepped up its efforts to address the health, housing, and social services needs of people with HIV/AIDS, homeless people have not benefitted as well as have domiciled people.

Finally, the chapter has presented evidence that opportunities for behavioral change and safe acts have resulted in successful education and prevention interventions with homeless HIV-infected people.

NOTES

1. Centers for Disease Control. *Summary of results—data from serosurveillance activities through 1991; 1992. Report on national HIV seroprevalence surveys.* 1992.

2. Luna, GC. *AIDS education and prevention.* Proceedings at the First International Conference on HIV and Homeless Youth: An Agenda for the Future. 1990.

3. Stricoff, RL, Kennedy, JT, Nattell, TC, Weisfuse, IB, and Novick, LF. HIV seroprevalence in a facility for runaway and homeless adolescents. *American Journal of Public Health*, 81, 1991, May, 50–53.

4. Rotherham-Borus, MJ, Koopman, C, Ehrhardt, AE. Homeless youths and HIV infection. *American Psychologist,* 46, 11, 1991, November, 1188–1196.

5. Barden, JC, Strife in families swells tide of homeless youths, *The New York Times*, February 5, 1990, A1, B8; and: Yates, G, MacKenzie, R, Pennbridge, J, and Cohen, E, A risk profile comparison of runaway and non-runaway youth. *American Journal of Public Health*, 1988, 820–821.

6. Robertson, MJ. Homeless youth in Hollywood: Patterns of alcohol use. Berkeley, CA: Alcohol Research Group; 1989.

7. Rotherham-Borus, Koopman, and Ehrhardt.

8. Rotherham-Borus, Koopman, and Ehrhardt; Yates, G, MacKenzie, R, Pennbridge, J, and Cohen, E. A risk profile comparison of runaway and non-runaway youth, *American Journal of Public Health*, 1988, 820–821, Hersch, P, Coming of age on city streets, *Psychology Today*, 1988, January, 28–36.

9. Harrigan, V. AIDS and the homeless: HIV prevention and care. In Land, H, (ed.), *AIDS: A Complete Guide to Intervention*. Milwaukee: Family Service America, Inc. 1992, 187–198.

10. County of Los Angeles. *HIV seroprevalence report for second quarter.* 1991; 1992.

11. Centers for Disease Control, 1992; and: King, D, Prostitutes as pariah in the age of AIDS: A content analysis of women prostitutes in the *New York Times* and the *Washington Post*, September 1985–April 1988, *Women and Health,* 16 (3–4), 155–176.

12. Wright, JD, *Address Unknown: The Homeless in America*. New York: Aldine de Gruyter; 1989, 61–67.

13. Centers for Disease Control, Division of Tuberculosis Control, Tuberculosis control among homeless populations, *Morbidity and Mortality Weekly Report*, 1987, 36, 257–260; and: Fackelmann, K, The double whammy of TB and AIDS, *Science News*, 1990, 137, 348.

14. Rosenthal, E. HIV infection thwarting efforts to detect TB and curb its spread. *The New York Times*, December 10, 1991, A1, B6.

15. Brickner, PW, Schaner, LK, Connan, B, Elvy, A, and Savage, M. *Health Care for Homeless People*. New York: Springer, 1985.

16. Institute for Medicine, Committee on Health Care for Homeless People. *Homeless, Health and Human Needs*, 1988.

17. Harrigan, 188.

18. Wright, JD, and Weber, E. *Homelessness and Health*. New York: McGraw Hill; 1987.

19. Harrigan, 192–194.

20. Lewis, CE. Primary care physicians refuse to care for HIV and other infected patients. *Western Journal of Medicine*, 156, January 12, 36–38.

21. Neely, M. AIDS and the homeless community. Testimony presented to the U.S. Senate Committee on Health and Human Services, December 17, 1991.

22. *Callahan et al.* v. *Carey et al.*, No. 42853/79, Supreme Court of the State of New York, 1979.

23. County of Los Angeles.

24. Pear, R. U.S. alters rules on people with HIV. *The New York Times*, December 17, 1991, A3.

25. Harrigan, 195.

26. Neely.

27. County of Los Angeles.

28. Homeless Health Care Los Angeles. Housing opportunities for persons with AIDS (HOPWA). *Health Care Monitor*, Winter 1993, 2, 2.

29. Savio, A. $7.2 million in HOPWA funds allocated to Los Angeles–Long Beach metropolitan region. *Homeless Reporter: Shelter Partnership*, April 1993, 4.

30. Kosterlitz, J. AIDS strains the system. *National Journal*, June 27, 1987. 1650–1654.

31. Brickner, P. *Health Care of Homeless People*. New York: Spring Publishing; 1985.

32. Lindblom, E. *Toward a Comprehensive Homeless Prevention Strategy*. Office of Housing Policy Research, Fannie Mae, Washington, DC, 1991.

33. Des Jarlais, DC, and Friedman, SR. The psychology of preventing AIDS among intravenous drug users: A social learning conceptualization. *American Psychologist*, 1991, 43, 865–870.

34. Rotherham-Borus, Koopman, and Ehrhardt.

35. Melia, N, Ford, WL, Kerndt, PR, Brown, ME, and Kelly, KE. Self-reported change in HIV associated risk behaviors in a homeless population. Presentation at 119th annual meeting of the American Public Health Association, 1991.

Chapter 10

Accessing an Understudied Population in Behavioral HIV/AIDS Research: Low-Income African-American Women

Robynn S. Battle
Gayle L. Cummings
Judith C. Barker
Flora M. Krasnovsky

INTRODUCTION

Limited studies exist examining behaviors in relation to human immunodeficiency virus (HIV) transmission among low-income African-American women outside of traditional high risk groups (Hahn, 1991; Rosenberg et al., 1992). Most studies conducted among low-income African-American women that have investigated HIV testing, sexual and behavioral characteristics, and prevalence of sero-positivity have focused on drug rehabilitation clients, sex industry workers, and clients from sexually transmitted disease (STD) or prenatal clinics (Corby et al., 1991; Gwinn et al., 1991; Lewis and Watters, 1989; Mays and Cocharan, 1988; CDC, 1992). These groups can be seen as captive audiences and somewhat more easily

This chapter was originally published in *Journal of Health and Social Policy*, Vol. 7(2) 1995.

The authors wish to thank the following individuals for their helpful comments: Patricia Saleba, MA; Virginia Nido, MA; Bonnie Faigeles, MA; Ralph DiClemente, PhD; and Donna Ford, BA.

This project is supported by a grant from the National Institute of Mental Health (Grant No. 2P50-MH42459).

accessible than women in the general population, such as homemakers and those who work in mainstream occupations. Low-income African-American women who do not fall into high-risk categories or who are not accessible through the previously mentioned sites are often considered to be "hard-to-reach" because of their ethnicity and socioeconomic status (SES) (Bowser, 1992; Freimuth and Mettger, 1990). This population may also be reluctant to participate in studies, based on their past experiences or knowledge of prior research projects (Jones, 1992; Thomas and Quinn, 1991).

The Parent Health Project studied a low-income African-American population. It was able to apply various approaches that actively gained the trust of the community, making this population more accessible. This chapter presents reasons why such communities are "hard-to-reach" and reports on a project that was successful at circumventing these problems. Discussed in this chapter will be the potential HIV transmission risk faced by African-American women; how certain methods and interpretation of data can misrepresent a community, leading to inefficient methods for data collection; and how methods and interpreted data can lead to barriers in recruitment or outreach. Finally, the Parent Health Project (PHP) and methods used to address the preceding issues will be presented. Concluding comments will discuss what PHP was able to learn through its alternative methods, and how the use of alternative methods may help in reaching "hard-to-reach" populations for behavioral AIDS research.

WOMEN AT RISK

Cases of acquired immune deficiency syndrome (AIDS) among women nationally have been on an increase in the last decade (Chu, Buehler, and Berkelman, 1990). While women made up 10.4% of all AIDS cases in 1988, they comprised 12.8% of all cases as of 1991 (Guinan, 1992). Among women's AIDS cases, African-American women have constituted 53% of reported cases, yet African-American women comprised only 17% of the total female population in the United States in 1990 (CDC, 1992). While it is estimated that HIV infection will continue to spread at a consistent rate among women, particularly among African-American women, studies of

HIV infection and behavior are still conducted mainly among traditional high-risk groups (Corby et al., 1991; Gwinn et al., 1991; Lewis and Watters, 1989; Mays and Cocharan, 1988).

HIV risk for women has often been measured in terms of multiple sexual partners, use of condoms, and having a sexual partner with an injection drug use or bisexual history (Berrios et al., 1992; Chu et al., 1992; Goldberg et al., 1992; Kim et al., 1993). However, women outside these risk categories may have other factors that place them at as much risk. For example, in the African-American community the high prevalence of STDs among crack-cocaine users creates HIV risk (Fullilove et al., 1990).

There is also an increasing concern about exposure to HIV infection through prisons. In a study of ten selected U.S. jails, and federal and state prisons, HIV seroprevalence was reported at 2.1% to 7.6% for men and 2.1% to 14.7% for women (Vlahov et al., 1991). Another study, conducted by the Justice Department, found that 30% of inmate deaths were attributed to AIDS; California ranked fourth in the nation among AIDS-related deaths among inmates. Estimates suggest that over 80% of injection drug users have served time in prison (CDC, 1990). Also, at any particular point in time, approximately one in four, or 25% of African-American men between the ages of 20 and 29 are under the supervision of the penal system (Russell, Wilson, and Hall, 1993). Given the risks of HIV transmission in prisons (CDC, 1992), the prevalence of persons with injection drug use history serving time (CDC, 1990; Vlahov et al., 1991), combined with the rate of African-American male inmates (Klein, Petersilia, and Turner, 1990), another possible risk arises for HIV transmission to African-American women. Women who are not injection drug users or who do not have a history of incarceration are at risk because of their partners' characteristics.

While HIV risk may be found in any community regardless of ethnic or socioeconomic level, it is still more prevalent in some African-American communities, and therefore increases the risk of people who do not fall within traditionally defined high-risk groups. This makes it more important to study people who have not been considered to be at risk, and to reevaluate factors that place them at risk.

RESEARCH ISSUES
IN THE AFRICAN-AMERICAN COMMUNITY

Studying a Community

As with any population being studied, there is concern about the information being gathered and the impact that the study results will have on the community (Weiss, 1977). This is especially true within the African-American community. If information is collected accurately but interpreted either incorrectly or inaccurately, this can lead to results that do not accurately depict the situation or population (Tsukashima, 1977; Weiss, 1977). For example, low usage of a medical facility in a community can be interpreted as the community not caring about its health, using it for only crisis situations, or simply not needing health care. What the low usage might actually indicate is that the facility is physically inaccessible to community members, operates at a time when people cannot get to it, or that many community members may feel uncomfortable in the facility.

In the case of HIV behavioral and sexual research, the issue of self-presentation and sexual disclosure within a community raises concern about how data is either collected or interpreted. Depending upon the interviewer and instrument design, data obtained may be inaccurate in relation to the studied community because of how it was collected or reported (Catania et al., 1990). Sometimes an instrument uses a word which has different meanings to the researcher and the participant. Such a word could be "sex," which can mean anything from kissing to vaginal intercourse. A question containing "sex" may or may not obtain the most accurate answer depending upon how it is interpreted by the interviewee. Other times, phrases or words are not probed by the interviewer. An example would be how a person responds to the question, "How does someone get AIDS?," and replies "Through sex." If left unprobed, the interviewer never knows exactly what is meant by "sex." To assume sex means vaginal sex could lead to misconceptions about the participant's level of understanding of AIDS or belittle the participant if the study takes the answer as a "simple answer" and assumes the participant knows little about AIDS. By using appropriate measures in interviews and instruments, the problem of accessing a community and then presenting inaccurate data can be alleviated.

In Weiss's (1977) assessment of research practices in community studies, 25% (n = 114) of the research groups surveyed preferred hiring indigenous individuals (persons with same ethnicity/race and socioeconomic status) as interviewers because it was felt that they alleviated suspicions about being studied and improved the validity of responses. Another 25% felt that involving the community helped in "drawing implications from the study's findings for future studies," and 11% felt that it "aided in interpreting the findings of the study." In comparison, 40% sought community involvement because they felt that community involvement promoted acceptance of their studies. Future research studies should strive to go beyond mere acceptance by a community and should involve it in the entire research process.

Questions have been raised by many researchers as to whether strategies such as hiring like interviewers (e.g., by ethnicity, gender, socioeconomic group), and being familiar with the community and subjects violate the validity of the study or produce subject bias (Blank et al., 1992). While these are concerns, with proper training of staff and good supervision during data collection, there is no need to assume that more error than usual will be introduced into the research process by such practices.

Some studies portray low-income and ethnic minority communities as powerless, apathetic, and isolated, leading to false assumptions and to misinformation which can further perpetuate discrimination, fallacy, and patronization (Freimuth and Mettger, 1990). Some assumptions are that African-American women are hard to reach (isolated), and that health concerns and worries are the same for both high- and low-risk women. Since most sexual behavior research has been conducted among middle-class white college students, it is not representative of all groups or subgroups in the population (Catania et al., 1990). Sexual behaviors among African-American women and their various subgroups have been understudied, and misrepresented and/or misunderstood, perhaps leading to research and health education efforts which fail or are ineffective.

For example, when an outpatient alcohol treatment model developed in Minnesota was implemented in a Swedish clinic, certain components of the program and the recruitment process did not apply to the Swedish patients due to cultural differences and perceptions of the program (Andreasson, Parmande, and Parmande, 1990). This finding was also echoed by researchers working with African-American women and obesity (Auslander et al., 1992; Kumanyika et al., 1991), and African Americans and behavioral change in general (Freudenberg, 1978). While behavioral change among all groups in a prevention program is the major goal, methods to induce behavioral change differ between African Americans and European Americans. Prevention programs that do not acknowledge salient social and cultural differences will result in understudying a population, misleading or erroneous interviews, and failing to prevent illness and death. Overlooking these differences limits the implementation of effective prevention programs to African-American women.

Barriers to Accessing the African-American Community

While false assumptions and misinterpretations perplex HIV behavioral research within the African-American community, these factors can in turn create barriers to accessing these populations. Two primary barriers to research within the African-American community have been identified as: African-American communities are "hard-to-reach"; and distrust from African Americans, as a result of their beliefs in theories of genocide and conspiracy.

It is often assumed that the African-American population is hard to reach. That this might be because they choose to remain so when attempts are made to study them is rarely considered (Bowser, 1992). When conducting research in any community on the effects of HIV infection or the factors that contribute to HIV transmission, the community's culture and perceptions of the disease must also be addressed (Bowser, 1992). Who or how individuals are recruited for a study, and the perceptions the studied group has about researchers, can determine the level of participation and the type of data the research team collects. A particular research methodology and type of recruitment may be efficient in one community and inefficient in others (Andreasson, Parmande, and Parmande, 1990).

Theories of genocide and conspiracy are held by many African Americans. These beliefs often translate into barriers to research in the African-American community. Such theories suggest drugs and certain incurable diseases, such as AIDS, were deliberately planted into the African-American community by the majority population in order to destroy the community (Page, 1992; Chinn, 1992; Thomas and Quinn, 1991). An often cited example is the Tuskegee Syphilis Study where African-American subjects were studied, yet preventive information and curative treatment was deliberately withheld (Caplan, 1992; Edgar, 1992; Jones, 1992; Thomas and Quinn, 1991). Other studies have shown that in certain community health programs people are reluctant to participate based on previous negative experiences with health workers and the program, such as lack of respect (Haynes, 1991). This and other misgivings within the African-American community lead individuals to believe that information will be used at the expense of the community, or not be used or shared with them. With HIV seroprevalence being disproportionately high among African Americans, the history of the Tuskegee study resurfaces as distrust by many African Americans for health authorities and research (Jones, 1992). These perceptions further foster the belief that there still exists the possibility of being exploited and abused in research, making people reluctant to participate (Haynes, 1991; Chinn, 1992).

Research Methodology

Existing methods and ideas about specific communities and AIDS may not be enough to understand the full impact of AIDS on the community. In order to assess adequately the needs of a population through research, it is necessary to incorporate methods which involve the community, yet obtain accurate data in gaining both descriptions about behaviors and about values and beliefs surrounding these behaviors within a community (Hahn, 1991).

While some health studies attempt to use community needs assessments in combination with survey research to make the most accurate assessments, others have simply applied survey research measures (Weiss, 1977). For example, some studies assess populations based on a survey alone, while other studies include field observations and community contact before implementing the survey (Tsukashima, 1977). Field observations may include focus groups and general (ethnographic) observations of the community as a whole. Community contact may include working through existing health or social services in the community such as a clinic, school district, or church (Auslander et al., 1992).

The Parent Health Project, described here, utilized both community involvement and survey method approaches. We believed it was important to conduct a study that would be both appropriate to the community and acceptable to health professionals and academia. We were willing to work on the issues of mistrust and misunderstanding so that they would not taint our research nor affect our presence in the community. The rest of this chapter looks at the various approaches that were taken in a behavioral health study to ensure accurate collection of information, to satisfy the community being studied, and "to give back" to the community based on study results.

PARENT HEALTH PROJECT

The Oakland Unified School District in conjunction with the University of California, San Francisco, conducted a study in an African-American population of elementary school children and their female caregivers: the Child Health Project (CHP) and Parent Health Project (PHP), where children ages five to 13, and their mothers or any female legal guardian who had raised the child, were interviewed to ascertain beliefs and concepts of health and disease processes, specifically AIDS. The purpose was to provide information so that comprehensive AIDS and disease prevention education programs could be developed for children and their adult caregivers. Furthermore, it was designed to gather critical information about: (1) a child and his or her female caregiver's concept of infectious diseases; (2) psychological and social correlates of disease concepts of the child and female caregiver; and (3) educational implications based upon children's and adults' understandings of the disease processes.

Both PHP and CHP reinforced links within a broad coalition that included the public school system, parent and community school leaders, community organizations, health professionals, and academic groups. The coalition consisted of health educators from the school district and county health services, principals of elementary schools, local community school workers, a psychologist, and public health educators. This coalition allowed the research team access into the community, which enabled the research team to gather the necessary information required for developing methods of teaching about communicable diseases and AIDS in a way that is culturally meaningful to African-American children and their parents/caregivers.

The project had an office in both the institutional home city and in the school district office in the city where the research project was being conducted. Using the school district office allowed us to build a rapport with the schools and be visible to district administrators.

The Research Process

Pilot Study. A pilot study enabled the team to examine issues and experiences that could either hinder or enhance the project, addressing the content of the research project, sample size, measurement tools, statistical tests, and the design of the research study itself. We were also able to address the context of the study, such as the social and cultural environment of study; the atmosphere of the interviewing area; the wording and response to certain questions; the day and time of the interviews; the times at which prospective interviewees were contacted; the rapport with the community, local schools, and community centers; and the impression each interviewee had of the project upon completion of the interview.

The pilot study highlighted certain components of the questionnaire which required rewording. For example, we found that the word "fat" generated for the adults many negative feelings toward the questions and the interview itself. When some women were asked questions such as, "How do you get fat?," "Do you worry about getting fat?," and "Do you think you are fat?," they became reluctant to talk, and shut down for the rest of the interview. Where possible, the word "fat" was changed to "overweight," thus taking away some of the negative connotations of "fat," and not offending the women. We knew we could lose valuable information by asking questions that caused parents/caregivers to be silent. By simply changing one word rather than the entire question we were able to obtain the amount and type of information needed for the study.

During the pilot study stages, PHP was also able to create strategies that ensured consistent and accurate data collection, and the building of rapport with the community. These strategies included team member/interviewer selection and the interview process.

Data Collection

Team Members. It was important to have team members who felt comfortable working within the particular community. Often, programs will select team members who are prepared academically, but underprepared to function outside of a standardized research environment. The PHP attempted to avoid this situation by creating a team with individuals who had academic research backgrounds, were experienced with and comfortable in working in the African-American community, and receptive of the community. Therefore they sought out interviewers who were: (1) women; (2) women around the same age as most of the mothers or who were mothers themselves; (3) African American; and (4) women with research backgrounds.

Team members also had to have the ability to understand what the parents/caregivers had to say both at an empathetic and linguistic level. There were times when the parents used terms with specific cultural meanings which required a particular response. For example, when an interviewee was discussing obesity, she talked about how she "couldn't hang with somebody who was fat because then I would get fat." While it may be interpreted as the interviewee viewing obesity as contagious, interviewers did not see this and understood her meaning. The interviewee meant that by being with someone (i.e., hanging) with the same social and eating patterns, she would be more inclined to eat and thus gain weight. For scoring answers, we needed team members who were able to adjust and understand these terms and the context in which the terms were used. This allowed us to get the most accurate information.

Interview Sites. We initially intended to conduct our interviews only at the child's school. We assumed it was an environment that would appear to be nonthreatening, safe, and comfortable due to its familiarity. However, this proved to be untrue; for security reasons the schools were often difficult to enter during school hours. Moreover, the days and hours we had selected proved to be inappropriate because many of the mothers worked. We had assumed that because we were in a community where over 80% of the families received Aid for Families with Dependent Children (AFDC), there would be no problem recruiting women to come for interviews on weekdays. Again, this proved to be untrue, since many mothers did have to work or had other obligations during the week. Through our local community contacts, we were able to set up and conduct our interviews at an additional site, a local youth community center that was easily accessible, safe, and provided a feeling of privacy. We also had the flexibility of scheduling appointments on Saturdays which was a more convenient time for many of the women.

The Instruments. Each selected mother/female caregiver underwent an individual, verbally administered, structured interview consisting of two components: a closed-ended demographic questionnaire designed to assess health history, sexual practices, and substance use; and an open-ended questionnaire designed to explore their concepts of health and disease including AIDS. The open-ended questionnaire was based on one developed at Harvard by Dr. David Schonfeld to assess children's concepts of health and illness and perceived vulnerability to illness (Schonfeld et al., 1993).

The Interview. An extra copy of the demographic questionnaire was given to the women to alleviate any discomfort or embarrassment from some of the more personal (drug and sexual history) questions. Since many of the answers were numbered, presenting an extra questionnaire allowed the women to answer with a number rather than stating the actual answer to the interviewer. For example, when inquiring about a woman's number of lifetime sex partners, the answers were categorized. When a woman answered, she could either verbally answer, read a categorized number, or point to the categorized number.

At the end of each interview, the women were asked if they had any questions regarding any information covered in the interview. Finally, they were given $50 for their time, along with a variety of brochures on topics such as AIDS, nutrition, and breast cancer screening.

During the reimbursement portion of the interview, interviewers also took the time to talk with the women about the interview process, and offer correct information for any of their incorrect responses, and to discuss any other topic that surfaced. It was during this time that women were allowed to express their feelings and concerns about themselves in relation to their health and social

environments. Responses were noted and then transcribed in a section of the survey called "Additional Comments." We felt that this
portion not only gave women a chance to talk about themselves,
giving us more insight into women's needs, but also allowed the
research team to perform a service for them. Health information
about HIV/AIDS and other health topics was provided. Referrals
were made for women who wanted things such as information about
special or accelerated education for their child; social services for
foster care or assistance; and sites for HIV testing. These discussions occurred at the end of the interview, and thus did not interfere
with or influence responses. It also made the research process less
threatening, and adhered to the community's needs. These "discussions" enabled us not only to get a better understanding of the
community, but also helped to establish credibility in the community when recruiting participants.

Recruiting Features

Initial Contact. While interviews took the form of verbal questionnaires and went through standard procedures for assuring confidentiality and informed consent, the team utilized various non-
standard approaches to contact participants. The purpose of the
recruitment was to get women to participate, as well as gain the
trust of the community (the school district and female caregivers).
Initially, our main contacts were gained through the school district
and the community outreach worker.

The Community Outreach Worker. Part of the new approach to
our research was to apply methods familiar in qualitative research
to standard survey procedures. These methods included a "grassroots" approach, such as working through a community outreach
worker. The person hired for the project had done outreach work in
the past for particular elementary schools in the area and was therefore familiar with children and their parents/caregivers, and with
issues such as mobility, changed phone numbers, and contact availability. Through the outreach worker, we were able to notify women
of the project occurring in their children's school and familiarize
them with the project. The outreach worker obtained names from
the school office, and contacted parents/female caregivers by phone
or in person. Because she was part of the community, she was able

to find out where families had moved and was able to locate mobile mothers. Upon locating the female caregivers, she was then able to perform a screening function, questioning them about demographics (family/child health history, financial and educational background), and to invite eligible women to be interviewed for the study. If the female caregiver agreed, an interview appointment was set up either by the outreach worker, or by one of the research team members.

The PHP took place after the child health study. We found, however, many women reluctant to sign up for interviews via the community workers. We concluded that women were uncomfortable having a community worker know that they were participating in a "sex study." While the community worker did familiarize the community and PHP with one another, the issue of sex carried a stigma which apparently made it difficult for the community worker to recruit women. After a year of working through the community outreach worker and establishing our reliability and trustworthiness, initial contact with parents was able to be done very successfully by team members via phone, referrals, and mail. Our previously established credentials made it possible to recruit women directly for the PHP.

Project Team Contact. The women were usually contacted by phone a week before the actual interview. Upon contact, the mother was informed about the purpose of the interview and monetary compensation, and invited to be interviewed. If she agreed to participate, she was given directions to the community center and the day and time of her interview. The contacting team member then sent out a follow-up letter, which included information about the interview and the interview date and time. A day before the interview, a team member contacted the female caregivers again, to remind them about the interviews. This strategy worked well and caught those who would be unable to attend, allowing the team to schedule other persons in their places.

Initially, we had hoped to select all participants randomly. Because of a high mobility rate (30%), we soon exhausted our list of eligible women, so we ended up also using referrals, thus adding ten subjects to our sample of 137 via referrals. We realized that many of the women were inaccessible via existing contact records, but were not unreachable if alternative methods, such as referrals, were used. Some female caregivers were referred to us by women who participated in the study. Others simply called to inquire after hearing about the study from a friend. Selection criteria still applied, and women recruited via referrals still had to have a child(ren) enrolled at one of the three study schools and be African American. Many times the women referred were women on the initial list whose phones were either disconnected or changed. At the end of their interviews, the women were asked if they knew other female caregivers who might be interested in being interviewed and how to contact these women. The women were also given two stamped flyers to give to other interested women who could fill out the flyers with their names and phone numbers and mail them back to the research team. With this information, women were contacted about being interviewed. Stamped flyers were also mailed to female caregivers of children at the participating schools, who were not interviewed for the Child Health Study. If interested, the women filled out the necessary information, and mailed the forms back to the research team. Altogether, we approached 200 women to request an interview, of whom 147 (74%) agreed to participate.

In conclusion, the PHP felt that it was necessary to work with people from within the community to establish initial contacts. We also worked with local community centers, and administrators from the schools to reinforce our intentions to collect information and share it with the community. Preliminary findings have been presented at a teachers' meeting in one of the study school sites, and future presentations to the school district are expected. By including people who were from and familiar with the community, and incorporating standard procedures to conduct research, the PHP was able to get better access to an understudied population. These relationships assisted the project in designing the recruitment and data collection components of our study.

DISCUSSION

The PHP had several objectives, one being the conduct of a feasible research project in a population that has been termed "difficult to reach." The team realized that this particular population was not necessarily unreachable, but perhaps reluctant to participate due to past histories of research in African-American communities and to women's present personal obligations to their families and work. We attempted to address both the communal and personal issues by making the project as flexible as possible to accommodate the needs of the women, yet retain scientific integrity.

Our study found that 22% of women had an existing sexual partner who had been in jail; 5% of the women reported having a partner who had been in jail for at least 12 months. This suggests that these ordinary African-American mothers/female caregivers may be facing additional risks with respect to HIV/AIDS that are not seen as risks by some researchers or health educators.

Rather than working solely as health researchers, we also took on the roles of health educators and community advocates. Through both roles we learned quite a bit about the community being studied and how further research and intervention projects in this particular community should be conducted.

Though we were unable to provide childcare, we set up appointments during times compatible with many of the mothers' schedules. During the interviews we listened to what the women felt were the issues that were bothering them. For many women, we found that HIV/AIDS was only one of several concerns that they felt they must deal with. Concerns about the health and welfare of their children, the possibility of getting off welfare, crime, and sometimes a sense of hopelessness were just a few of the concurrent issues they were also dealing with.

"Hard-to-reach" is the term that has been used to describe our target group of low-income African-American women. The concept "hard-to-reach" poses the following questions: (1) Is the group "hard-to-reach" because they choose to be? Is it reluctant to participate, making it "hard" to recruit them? and (2) Do the research instruments provide an in-depth measurement of group social and cultural factors which influence or hinder behavioral change? Do they limit the type of data collected, or measure only certain behaviors, associations and correlations, leaving out anyone who does not fit stereotypical categories (e.g., bisexual partner or IV drug using partner)?

Through our planning and recruitment efforts, we found that our target group was "hard-to-reach" only when "traditional" public health survey research methodologies were used, such as recruitment in STD or health clinics or with the use of standard closed-ended questionnaires. Sometimes these traditional research methodologies fail to recognize the impact of race, culture, gender, and socioeconomic status, thus limiting who is recruited and the information collected. Studies which do not consider these issues not only create barriers to access, but "fatally flaw their . . . interpretation of data" (Rosnow, 1993). Lack of recognition of cultural and other differences not only sets limits on the interpretation of data but also covers up any implications that the data may have about an individual's or group's behaviors in relation to HIV transmission (Nelkin et al., 1990; Singer, 1992; Stall, 1993).

A community's culture and their perceptions of research must also be considered when conducting research. Some behavioral health researchers assume that people are readily available for study or want to be studied. This is not always the case (Bowser, 1992). To overlook a community's attitudes, concerns, and issues about how it responds to a research study or intervention program not only produces difficulty in recruiting a community's participation but also confounds the collected data. Sometimes the urgency of addressing a health problem in a community (such as AIDS, infant mortality, cancer, or hypertension) overshadows the attitudes of those being studied, eventually driving participants away so that they are "hard to reach," reluctant to participate in a study, and feel they are not respected.

In reviewing the efforts of HIV/AIDS intervention programs, Choi and Coates (1993) found that many programs produced short-term behavioral change among participants, yet long-term outcome was not significant. With the HIV/AIDS epidemic entering its second decade, research must now study not only people's behaviors, but the context in which they occur, and what will elicit change in both the short and long terms. To do this, research studies will need to incorporate investigation of "other" issues, such as housing, economics, parental status, and living situations, and to examine how these issues influence a person's behavior or willingness or ability to change behavior. Several studies around the world are using both qualitative or ethnographic techniques in addition to quantitative methods to measure and assess people's sexual behaviors in context, investigate contextual issues such as sources of income, religion, perceived gender roles in a culture, and cultural or ethnic identity (Asha, 1993; Mmari, 1993; Cash and Anasuchaktkul, 1993; Singer, 1992; Flaskerud and Nyamathi, 1990; Williams et al., 1988). Studies in the United States, too, must use instruments that investigate and measure contextual issues.

In addition to conceptual focus change, methods will also have to alter. Broadening notions of eligibility for participation in research studies must include, for example, different recruitment sites (e.g., other than a hospital, STD or prenatal clinics). Interventions, though theoretically grounded, may have to involve a community service to administer or even design an appropriate intervention. Only through these methods will studies be able to determine what factors influence sexual behavioral change. Through highly interactive activities and peer support groups, research will be able to find out what interventions work well and address particular sexual behaviors. Research studies must involve the community being studied, as well as develop ways to recruit and obtain data that represents the full diversity of the population. This may require: a community needs assessment which, although time-consuming, is important; community and study population focus groups; and, the adjustment of an in-progress research protocol. With the need for further understanding of people's behaviors in relation to behavior change and HIV/AIDS, behavioral research must move in a direction that does not alienate people or continuously create "hard-to-reach" populations.

BIBLIOGRAPHY

Andreasson, S, Parmande, M, and Parmande, SP. A Trial That Failed, and the Reasons Why: Comparing the Minnesota Model with Outpatient Treatment and Non-Treatment for Alcohol Disorders. *Scandinavian Journal of Social Medicine*, 1990; 18: 221–224.

Asha, K. Cultural and Socio/Economic Factors as an Impediment to HIV Prevention Among Rural Women in Trinidad and Tobago. IXth International Conference on AIDS, Berlin, 1993.

Auslander, WF, Haire-Joshua, D, Houston, CA, and Fisher, EB. Community Organization to Reduce the Risk of Non-Insulin-Dependent Diabetes Among Low-Income African-American Women. *Ethnicity and Disease*, 1992; 2: 177–184.

Berrios, DC, Hearst, N, Perkins, LL et al. HIV Antibody Testing in Young, Urban Adults. *Archives of Internal Medicine*, 1992; 152: 397–402.

Blank, PD, Bellack, AS, Rosnow, RL et al. Scientific Rewards and Conflicts of Ethical Choices in Human Subjects Research. *American Psychologist*, 1992; 47(7): 959–965.

Bowser, BP. African-American Culture and AIDS Prevention: From Barrier to Ally. *Western Journal of Medicine*, 1992; 157(3): 286–289.

Caplan, AL. When Evil Intrudes. Hastings Center Report. 1992; 22(6): 29–32.

Cash, K ,and Anasuchaktkul, B. Relevant AIDS Education for Thai Adolescent Female Workers. IXth International Conference on AIDS, Berlin, 1993.

Catania, JA, Gibson, GR, Chitwood, DD, and Coates, TJ. Methodological Problems in AIDS Behavioral Research: Influences on Measurement Error and Participation Bias in Studies of Sexual Behavior. Psychological Bulletin. 1990; 108(3): 339–362.

Center for Disease Control. HIV Prevention in the U.S. Correctional System, 1991. MMWR. 1992; 41(22): 389–381 and 397.

Center for Disease Control. HIV/AIDS Surveillance Report. U. S. AIDS Cases Reported through September 1992. U. S. Department of Health and Human Services. 1992: 8–10.

Center for Disease Control. Risk Behaviors for HIV Transmission Among Intravenous Drug Users Not in Drug Treatment—U.S. 1987–1989. MMWR. 1990; 39: 273–276.

Center for Disease Control. Tuberculosis Morbidity—United States, 1992. MMWR. 1993; 42(18): 363.

Chinn, JC. Remember Tuskegee. *New York Times* 29, May 1992.

Choi, K, and Coates, TJ. What Does the Empirical Literature Say About Programs, Outcomes, Implications, and Research Directions? In Review.

Chu, SY, Buehler, JW, and Berkelman, RL. Impact of the Human Immunodeficiency Virus Epidemic on Mortality in Women of Reproductive Age, United States. Journal of the American Medical Association. 1990; 264 (2): 225–229.

Chu, SY, Peterman, TA, Doll, LS et al. AIDS in Bisexual Men in the United States: Epidemiology and Transmission to Women. American Journal of Public Health. 1992; 82(2): 224–229.

Corby, NH, Wolitski, MA, Thornton-Johnson, S et al. AIDS knowledge, Perception of Risk and Behaviors Among Female Sex Partners of Injection Drug Users. AIDS Education and Prevention. 1991; 9(2): 92–95.

Edgar, H. Outside the Community. Hastings Center Report. 1992; 22(6): 32–35.

Flaskerud, JH, and Nyamathi, AM. Effects of an AIDS Education Program on the Knowledge, Attitudes, and Practices of Low Income Black and Latina Women. Journal of Community Health. 1990; 14(6): 343–355.

Freimuth, VS, and Mettger, W. Is There a Hard-To-Reach Audience? Public Health Reports. 1990; 105(3): 232–238.

Freudenberg, N. Shaping the Future of Health Education: From Behavior Change to Social Change. Health Education Monogram. 1978; 6: 373–377.

Fullilove, RE, Fullilove, MT, Bowser, B et al. Crack Users: The New AIDS Risk Group? Cancer Detection and Prevention. 1990; 14: 363–367.

Goldberg, DJ, Emslie, JA, Smyth, Reid, D et al. A System for Surveillance of Voluntary HIV Testing: Results of the First Two Years, 1989–1990. AIDS. 1992; 6(5): 495–500.

Guinan, ME. HIV, Heterosexual Transmission, and Women. Journal of the American Medical Association. 1992; 268(4): 520–521.

Gwinn, M, Pappaionou, M, George, JR et al. Prevalence of HIV Infection in Child-bearing Women in the U.S. Journal of the American Medical Association. 1991; 265: 1704–1708.

Hahn, RA. What Should Behavioral Scientists Be Doing About AIDS? Social Science and Medicine. 1991; 33(1): 1–3.

Haynes, MA. Making Cancer Prevention Effective for African Americans. Statistical Bulletin. 1991; 18–21.

Holmes, KK, Karon, JM, and Kreiss, J. The Increasing Frequency of Heterosexually Acquired AIDS in the United States, 1983–88. American Journal of Public Health. 1990; 80(7): 858–862.

Jones, JH. The Tuskegee Legacy: AIDS and the Black Community. Hastings Center Report. 1992; 22(6): 38–40.

Kim, MY, Marmor, M, Neil, D, and Wolfe, H. HIV Risk-Related Sexual Behaviors Among Heterosexuals in New York City: Associations with Race, Sex, and Intravenous Drug Use. AIDS. 1993; 7(3): 409–414.

King, PA. The Dangers of Difference. Hastings Center Report. 1992; 22(6): 35–38.

Klein, S, Petersilia, J, and Turner, S. Race and Imprisonment Decisions in California. Science. 1990; 47: 812–816.

Kumanyika, SD, Obarnaneck, E, Stevens, VJ et al. Weight-loss Experience of Black and White Participants in NHLBI-Sponsored Clinical Trials. American Journal of Clinical Nutrition. 1991; 53: 1631S–1638S.

Lewis, DK, and Watters, JK. Human Immunodeficiency Virus Seroprevalance in Female Intravenous Drug Users: The Puzzle of Black Women's Risk. Social Science Medicine. 1989; 29: 1071–1075.

Mays, VM, and Cocharan, SD. Issues in the Perception of AIDS Risk Reduction Activities by Black and Hispanic/Latina Women. American Psychologist. 1988; 43: 949–957.

Mmari, VJ. Women in Developing Countries: The Case Study of Economic Factors as a Function of HIV Sexual and Behavioral Risks Among African Women. IXth International Conference on AIDS, Berlin, 1993.

Nelkin D, Willis D and Parris S. Introduction. Milbank Memorial Fund Quarterly. 1990; 68: 1–9.

Page, C. Black Rage and Conspiracy Theories. Emerge. 1992; 3(5): 43 and 45.

Rosenberg, PS, Levy, ME, Brundage, JF et al. Population-Based Monitoring of an Urban HIV/AIDS Epidemic: Magnitude and Trends in the District of Columbia. Journal of the American Medical Association. 1992; 268(4): 495–503.

Rosnow, RL. The Volunteer Problem Revisited. In PD Blank, Interpersonal Expectations: Theory, Research, Applications. 1993. New York, Cambridge University Press.

Russell, KY, Wilson, M, and Hall, RE. Color Complex: The Politics of Skin Color Among African Americans. Harcourt Brace Jovanovich, Inc. 1993. New York, NY. US.

Schonfeld, DJ, Johnson, SR, Perrin, EC, O'Hare, LL, and Ciccheti, DV. Understanding of Acquired Immune-Deficiency Syndrome by Elementary School Children—A Developmental Survey. Pediatrics. 1993; 92(3): 385–389.

Singer, M. AIDS and US Ethnic Minorities: The Crisis and Alternative Anthropological Responses. Human Organization. 1992; 51(1): 89–95.

Stall, R. Alcohol and Drug Use and AIDS: The Uses of Anthropology. Paper presented to the American Anthropological Association, New Orleans. 1993.

Thomas, SB, and Quinn, SC. The Tuskegee Syphilis Study, 1932 to 1972: Implications for HIV Education and AIDS Risk Education Programs in the Black Community. American Journal of Public Health. 1991; 81: 1498–1504.

Tsukashima, RT. Merging Fieldwork and Survey Research in the Study of a Minority Community. Journal of Social Issues. 1977; 33(4): 133–143.

Vlahov, D, Brewer, TF, Castro, KG et al. Prevalence of Antibody to HIV-1 Among Entrants to U. S. Correctional Facilities. Journal of the American Medical Association. 1991; 265: 1129–1132.

Weiss, C. Survey Researchers and Minority Communities. Journal of Social Issues. 1977; 33(4): 20–35.

Williams, DE, Vitiello, MV, Reis, RK et al. Successful Recruitment of Elderly Community-Dwelling Subjects for Alzheimer's Disease Research. Journal of Gerontology: Medical Sciences. 1988; 43(3): M69–74.

Chapter 11

Access to Primary Care Among Young African-American Children in Chicago

Michele A. Kelley
Janet D. Perloff
Naomi M. Morris
Wangyue Liu

INTRODUCTION

Black children experience greater mortality and morbidity than their white counterparts. In 1989, the black infant mortality rate (IMR) was 18.6, more than twice the white IMR of 8.1 (National Center for Health Statistics, 1990). Black children (under age 18) are more than twice as likely (4.8%) as their Caucasian counterparts (2.1%) to have self-reported health status as "fair" or "poor" (rather than excellent or good) (National Center for Health Statistics, 1990). Similarly, black children with chronic illnesses are more likely to experience limitations of activity (inability to participate in or perform in age-appropriate play, educational activities or self-care) than nonblack children (5.6% v. 5.0%) (National Center for Health Statistics, 1990).

Racial differentials exist in overall use of health care services. For children under five years of age, whites had a mean of 7.6 visits per year, while black children had 4.6 visits (National Center for

This chapter was originally published in *Journal of Health & Social Policy*, Vol. 5(2) 1993.

Health Statistics, 1989). For physician visits for routine (preventive) care, the 1988 National Health Interview Survey (HIS-child health supplement) found no overall racial differences in likelihood of at least one visit for preventive care. Approximately 64% of all children under 18 years of age had at least one preventive visit. However, significant racial differences emerged by age, with the greatest differential observed among infants. Among white infants, 95.1% had a physician visit for routine care, while only 87.6% of black infants had a routine visit. When access to a regular source of care is considered for children under age 18, no racial differences were observed, with approximately 88% of all children having a source of care. However, significant racial differences exist among younger children with the greatest disparity among infants. The percentage of black infants with a regular source of care was 79.8%, compared with white infants at 92.1% (Bloom, 1990).

The type of facility in which care is received varies by race and other socio-demographic factors. The HIS found that black children were three times more likely (35%) than white children (11%) to receive care in "institutional" settings, that is, hospital-based clinics, health departments, or nonprofit community health centers. Regardless of race, children residing in inner cities were more likely (23%) to receive care in these institutional settings compared to suburban (11%) or rural children (16%). Infants residing in the inner city were particularly more likely (33%) to receive care in such facilities than suburban infants (16%) or infants in rural areas (16%) (Bloom, 1990).

In summary, there is substantial evidence that while black children have increased morbidity, they also have fewer visits to physicians (National Center for Health Statistics, 1990). These differentials in health status and access to care are strongly associated with socio-economic status (Egbuonu and Starfield, 1982; Newacheck and Starfield, 1988). Although the federal Medicaid program has reduced financial barriers to access to care (Gortmacher, 1981; Rosenbach, 1989), less than 44% of low-income black children (living in families below 200% of the poverty level) are covered by Medicaid (Children's Defense Fund, 1989). Black children living with an employed family member are also more likely (29.3%) than white children (17.5%) to lack any type of health insurance coverage (Children's Defense Fund, 1989).

Recently, the U.S. Public Health Service has adopted overall goals to decrease disparities in health status and access to primary care, with special emphasis on children (Public Health Service, 1990). In order for local communities to achieve these goals, information on current patterns of care arrangements and care use must be obtained (American Public Health Association, 1991).

This chapter will present results of a study of access to care among young African-American children (under age six) residing in three high-risk communities in Chicago. Two general questions guided our analyses:

Among young African-American children residing in high-risk communities in Chicago,

1. What factors are associated with having an identified regular source of care?
2. What health care arrangements are used for illness and preventive care?

Findings have implications for child health policy and services research in the inner city, especially given the recent expansion of Medicaid to include children up to age six years of age in households with incomes up to 133% of the federal poverty level (Omnibus Budget Reconciliation Act, 1989).

METHODS

Maternal respondents were black, age 18 to 44, residing in three low-income communities in Chicago with high infant mortality rates: the Near West Side, West Garfield Park, and Austin. Each of these community areas in Chicago's west side is at least 70% African-American and each is designated as a "high-risk" area for maternal and child health (Chicago Department of Health, 1990), with an overall infant mortality rate of 20.9 (per 1,000 live births) in 1988, nearly twice the national target rate of 11 for black infants (Public Health Service, 1990).

Respondents were part of a study designed to examine access to maternal and child health care. Data were obtained from a cross-sectional survey conducted by the authors during the fall of 1989. Technical expertise for the sampling design, instrument development, and data collection was provided to the authors' specifications under a contract with the University of Illinois Survey Research Laboratory (SRL). Interviews were conducted by black females trained and supervised by SRL.

A two-stage sampling method was used. First, census tracts were randomly selected from among those in the lowest two quartiles of household income as indicated in the 1980 census. Then blocks were randomly selected from within the selected tracts. Respondents were eligible to be interviewed in their homes if they were black, between the ages of 18 and 44, and were either pregnant at the time of the interview or had a child under six years of age in the home. Subjects were identified by door-to-door screening. Total cooperation, i.e., with both screening and completed interview, was 87.7%. A total of 305 women were interviewed. Nine women were excluded as they had no children under age six, yielding a final sample size of 296.

Measures

The questionnaire measured sociodemographic characteristics, self-reported health status, pregnancy history, and health care access and use of each woman and her youngest child. Items were adapted from the widely used National Health Interview Survey core questionnaire and 1988 child health supplement (National Center for Health Statistics, 1989). To reduce the possibility of misclassification error in the dependent variable, subjects were asked both the name and address of the place that they usually used for ambulatory (nonemergent) care and for preventive care (if different) for themselves and for their children. This information was then verified using local medical provider listings and site visits to assign the appropriate facility type: office-based physician, hospital ER/OPD, nonprofit community clinic, or health department clinic.

RESULTS

Characteristics of the sample are presented in Table 11.1. Although 62% of the women had completed 12 or more years of

TABLE 11.1. Association of Demographic and Economic Factors with Access to Child Health Care

	Child Has a Regular Source of Care				
	yes		no		
	n	(%)	n	(%)	p[a]
Maternal age					NS
18-29	195	(67.94)	14	(4.88)	
30-44	73	(25.44)	5	(1.74)	
Marital status					NS
now married	53	(18.03)	1	(0.34)	
not married	222	(75.51)	18	(6.12)	
Education					NS
< 12th grade	102	(34.90)	10	(3.40)	
≥ 12th grade	173	(58.84)	9	(3.06)	
Family structure					NS
woman alone	133	(45.08)	12	(4.07)	
with other adult	143	(48.47)	7	(2.37)	

TABLE 11.1 (continued)

| | Child Has a Regular Source of Care | | | | p^a |
| | yes | | no | | |
	n	(%)	n	(%)	
AFDC[b]					
yes	186	(63.27)	15	(5.10)	NS
no	89	(30.27)	4	(1.36)	
Medicaid					
yes	205	(69.26)	16	(5.41)	NS
no	72	(24.32)	3'	(1.01)	
Labor force					
employed	77	(26.19)	1	(0.34)	*
unemployed	198	(67.35)	18	(6.12)	
Years lived in community					
< 5 years	122	(41.36)	13	(4.41)	*
≥ 5 years	154	(52.20)	2	(2.03)	
Child age					
infant	74	(25.00)	10	(3.38)	*
1 to 5 years	203	(68.58)	9	(3.04)	

[a] Using the χ^1 test of significance: *df* =1
* p < .05
** p < .01
[b] Family receives benefits from the Aid to Families with Dependent Children program.

education, the majority were unmarried (81.6%) and about one-half lived in households with no other adult present. Over two-thirds were receiving benefits from the Aid to Families with Dependent Children program and about three-fourths were enrolled in Medicaid. When Medicaid and other sources of insurance were combined, 90% of respondents had some form of insurance coverage. Just over one-fourth of the women were employed at least part time. The median age of the women in the sample was 26 years. Approximately 28% of children were infants. The median age of the youngest child was 24 months.

Access to Care

Overall, 93.6% of children in the sample had a regular source of care, that is, an identifiable facility for acute illness care. Almost two-thirds (62.4%) of mothers reported that they used the same place for their children's care as for their own care. These mothers tended to be less educated ($\chi^2 = 2.80$; df $= 1$; p $< .10$) and more worried about their child's health ($\chi^2 = 3.10$; df $= 1$; p $< .10$). Approximately 88% indicated they had a usual place for well-child care, that is, for recommended check-ups and immunizations when their children were well. Infants were less likely than older children (17.9% v. 10%) to have a place for well-child care ($\chi^2 = 3.50$; df $= 1$; p $< .10$). Overall, 95% of mothers reported that their children had a well-child visit within the past year. Ninety percent used the same place for both preventive and illness care. Infants were more likely than other children to use the same place ($\chi^2 = 3.37$; df $= 1$; p $< .10$).

Table 11.1 presents selected demographic and economic factors as associated with having a regular source of care. Maternal employment, length of time in the community, and having a child older than age one were positively associated with having access to child health care. In Table 11.2, neither self-reported measures of maternal health status nor maternal perceptions of child health status were associated with access to child health care. However, mothers who themselves had a regular source of care were more likely to have access to care for their youngest children.

TABLE 11.2. Association of Self-Reported Health Status and Maternal Access to Care with Access to Child Health Care

| | Child Has a Regular Source of Care | | | | |
| | yes | | no | | |
	n	(%)	n	(%)	p[a]
Maternal health					
excellent/good	228	(77.29)	13	(4.41)	NS
fair/poor	48	(16.27)	6	(2.03)	
Mother now pregnant					
yes	25	(8.47)	3	(1.02)	NS
no	251	(85.08)	16	(5.42)	
Maternal chronic illness[b]					
yes	57	(19.26)	2	(0.68)	NS
no	220	(74.32)	17	(5.74)	

TABLE 11.2 (continued)

| | Child Has a Regular Source of Care | | | | |
| | yes | | no | | p^a |
	n	(%)	n	(%)	
Mother has regular source of care					
yes	254	(85.81)	13	(4.39)	**
no	23	(7.77)	6	(2.03)	
Child health					
excellent/good	251	(84.80)	17	(5.74)	NS
fair/poor	26	(8.78)	2	(0.68)	
Comparable child health					
better/same	261	(89.69)	19	(6.53)	NS
worse	11	(3.78)	0	(0.00)	
Concern about child health[c]					
worried	85	(28.72)	7	(2.36)	NS
not worried	192	(64.86)	12	(4.05)	

a Using the χ^2 test of significance: $df = 1$

** $p < .01$

b Diabetes, hypertension, asthma, or any condition requiring regular medication

c Mothers were asked to compare youngest child's health with the health of other children the same age.

Care Arrangements

The usual source of child health care by facility type is presented in Table 11.3. The majority of children used private office-based physicians, followed by hospital-based clinics and nonprofit community clinics. In these analyses, we have collapsed federally funded neighborhood health centers and local health department clinics into the nonprofit community clinic category. This category excludes ambulatory care facilities associated with community hospitals. We explored factors associated with use of child health facility type. In general, particular attributes of primary care and respondent characteristics differentiated those who used community clinics from either office-based physicians or hospital-based clinics.

Compared with the other two facility types, mothers were more likely to report ability to receive advice by telephone from community clinics ($\chi^2 = 4.74$; df = 2; p < .10). Those who used community clinics for their children's care were more likely to report seeing one particular provider (provider continuity) ($\chi^2 = 16.41$; df = 2; p < .001). Mothers using community clinics were least likely to be worried about their children's health, while those using hospitals were more likely to worry ($\chi^2 = 6.40$; df = 2; p < .05). Additionally, mothers who used community clinics were more likely to have lived in the community for five or more years ($\chi^2 = 5.75$; df = 2; p < .10), or to have completed high school ($\chi^2 = 5.42$; df = 2 p < .10), or to have at least one other adult living in the household ($\chi^2 = 7.56$; df = 2; p < .05).

TABLE 11.3. Usual Source of Child Health Care Facility Type[a]

	n	(%)
Private office	140	(47.6)
Hospital-based facility	85	(28.9)
Nonprofit community clinic[b]	50	(17.0)
No particular place	19	(6.5)

[a] Two responses could not be classified and are considered missing data.
[b] Includes local health department clinics.

In addition to increased telephone access, virtually all of the children who used community clinics for their regular sources of illness care used the same place for their preventive care. Although information on maternal satisfaction with child health care received was not obtained, mothers who used community clinics for their children's care were more likely to be satisfied with their own care ($\chi^2 = 7.13$; df = 2; p < .05). Furthermore, these community clinic users were more likely to rate the quality of child health care available in their neighborhoods as "excellent or good" than those who used either of the other two facility types ($\chi^2 = 5.43$; df = 2; p < .10).

DISCUSSION

Few demographic and economic and health status factors in this study were associated with access to care. These results, which differ from findings in major multivariate studies, may be explained in part by the relatively homogeneous population. Findings that maternal employment and length of residence in the community were positively associated with having a regular source of care may represent the effects of social integration, through which mothers may gain information about pediatric care. The influence of social networks on pediatric use remains largely unexplored and holds promise as a factor in the design of community-based child health promotion programs.

The finding that almost 18% of infants lacked a source of preventive care and that this age group was less likely than older children to have a preventive care source was striking, given national priorities for reduction of infant mortality and promoting healthy development over the first year of life (Public Health Service, 1989). These findings parallel results of the recent National Health Interview Survey which found that over 10% of infants lacked a source of preventive care and this age group was least likely among children under age eight to have a source of preventive care. Preventive or "well-child" care is especially important given the opportunities it affords for early detection of health problems, anticipatory guidance, and immunizations. A recent study by the Centers for Disease Control found that less than 28% of two-year-olds in Chicago were appropriately immunized (Centers for Disease Control, 1991). The implications for action are clear: women and their newborn infants must be linked with an accessible source of pediatric care before hospital discharge.

Approximately one-half (50.9%) of children in this sample who had a regular source of care used private physicians. However, children who used community clinics (18.2%), e.g., health department clinics and other nonprofit community clinics, appeared to have more optimal care arrangements. That is, they experienced more continuity by receiving preventive and illness care at the same place, and seeing the same provider. Additionally, mothers of children seen in these clinic settings were more likely to have telephone contact with their providers, an important component of pediatric care which encourages appropriate utilization, fosters compliance, provides opportunities for anticipatory guidance, and increases parental satisfaction with care (American Academy of Pediatrics, 1991; Kelley, 1988).

Although quality of care received was not measured directly in this study, maternal perception of quality of child health care available in local neighborhoods was higher among clinic users. There is evidence to suggest that some private physicians serving large numbers of Medicaid patients in the innercity may provide care of a less technical quality (Handler, Perloff, and Kennelly, 1992). Additionally, these providers typically do not practice with a multidisciplinary health care team, nor are they as likely to be formally linked to other health and social services in the community through comprehensive service networks (Brown, 1988).

Case-management services to enable children and their families to access services in the community could enhance the scope of care provided in private office settings. Research is needed to examine the feasibility of engaging office-based providers into comprehensive service networks, and to compare the effectiveness of these enhanced office-based services with "institutional" settings relative to child health status measures and access to care. Such research is important and timely in light of the new federal *Healthy Start* initiative, which will provide care to women and infants in 15 urban and rural target communities, with an emphasis on comprehensive service networks (Federal Register, 1991).

REFERENCES

American Academy of Pediatrics, Committee on Practice and Ambulatory Medicine (1991). The office telephone triage training and technique. In L.A. Kutnik, E.J. Saltzman, D.W. Shea, L.S. Honigfeld and K.S. Palchick (eds.), *Management of Pediatric Practice, 2nd edition.* Elk Grove Village, IL, 38–46.

American Public Health Association (1991). *Healthy communities 2000: Model standards,* 3rd edition. Washington, DC.

Bloom, B. (1990). *Health insurance and medical care: Health of our nation's children, U.S., 1988.* Advance data from vital and health statistics; no. 188. Hyattsville, MD: National Center for Health Statistics.

Brown, S.S. (ed.) (1988). *Prenatal care: Reaching mothers, reaching infants.* Washington, DC: National Academy Press.

Centers for Disease Control (1991). *Retrospective immunization status assessment based on a review of school health records of kindergarten children in public schools in Chicago: Final report.* Atlanta, GA.

Chicago Department of Health (1990). *Chicago and Cook County health care action plan: Report of the Chicago and Cook County health care summit* (vol. 2). Chicago: Chicago Department of Health.

Children's Defense Fund (1989). *A vision for America's future.* Washington, DC.

Egbuonu, L., and Starfield, B. (1982). Child health and social status. *Pediatrics,* 69, 550–557.

Federal Register (1991). *Healthy Start Initiative* (56) 74. (April 27, 1991), Washington, DC: U.S. Department of Health and Human Services.

Gortmacher, S.L. (1981). Medicaid and the Health Care of Children in Poverty and Near Poverty. *Medical Care,* 19, 567–582.

Handler, A., Perloff, J., and Kennelly, J.B. (1992). Ensuring the quality of maternity care. In J. Kotch, C.H. Blakely, S.S. Braun, and F.Y. Wong (eds.), *A pound of prevention: The case for universal maternity care in the U.S.* Washington, DC: American Public Health Association, 223–251.

Kelley, M.A. (1988). Maternal satisfaction with primary care for children with selected chronic conditions (Doctoral dissertation, Johns Hopkins University).

National Center for Health Statistics (1989). *Current estimates from the national health interview survey, 1988.* Vital and Health Statistics (10) 173. Hyattsville, MD.

National Center for Health Statistics (1990). Health of black and white Americans, 1985–87. Vital and health statistics (10) 171. Hyattsville, MD.

Newacheck, P.W., and Starfield, B. (1988). Morbidity and use of ambulatory care services among poor and nonpoor children. *American Journal of Public Health,* 78, 927–933.

Omnibus Budget Reconciliation Act (1989). Public Law 101–239, Section 6401 *"Mandatory coverage of certain low income women and children"* (December 19, 1989).

Public Health Service (1989). *Caring for our future: The content of prenatal care.* Washington, DC.

Public Health Service (1990). *Healthy children 2000: National health promotion and disease prevention objectives related to mothers, infants, children, adolescents and youth.* Washington, DC: U.S. Government Printing Office, DHHS Publication No. HRSA-M-CH 91–2.

Rosenbach, M.L. (1989). The impact of Medicaid on physician use by low-income children. *American Journal of Public Health,* 79, 1220–1226.

Chapter 12

High Risk Channeling to Improve Medicaid Maternal and Infant Care

Samuel L. Baker
Jennie J. Kronenfeld

To improve the medical care access of the poorest women and newborns, South Carolina began a High Risk Channeling Project in April 1986. The Project directs physicians to screen all Medicaid-eligible pregnant women and newborns for specified clinical high risk factors. High risk patients are channeled to designated clinics for prenatal and newborn care. Channeled pregnant women are directed to deliver their babies at regional referral hospitals.

For the first two years of the Project, about two-thirds of pregnancies and 60% of newborns were actually screened. Channeled women were much more likely than the nonchanneled to deliver at higher level hospitals. In counties where relatively few women were channeled, the rate of prematurity among Medicaid newborns was significantly higher than in other counties.

To improve the medical care access of the poorest women and newborns, South Carolina has operated its High Risk Channeling Project since April 1986. The Project requires physicians to screen all Medicaid-eligible pregnant women and newborns for specified clinical high risk factors. High risk patients are channeled to designated clinics, with board-certified specialist physicians on staff, for prenatal and newborn care. At the clinics, patients also receive social work and nutritional counseling. The clinics provide active

This chapter was originally published in *Journal of Health & Social Policy*, Vol. 3(4) 1992.

follow-up, and an examination one year after the initial visit. High risk pregnant women are directed to deliver their babies at regional Level II or III hospitals.

The High Risk Channeling Project is conducted under a formal waiver of the patients' freedom of choice of provider. The Health Care Financing Administration (HCFA), the federal agency responsible for Medicaid, granted the waiver for the Project to begin in 1986, and has renewed the waiver after reviews in 1988 and 1990. A condition of the waiver renewals has been that the Project improve access and outcomes, with consequent net savings of Medicaid costs.

The data sources available for investigating the effectiveness of the High Risk Channeling Project were: Medicaid bills from hospitals and physicians for all deliveries and newborns, whether in the Project or not; databases of screening forms, maintained by the Office of High Risk Care of the South Carolina state Medicaid agency, the State Health and Human Services Finance Commission, and a database of High Risk Clinic care recipients, maintained by the South Carolina Department of Health and Environmental Control. Unfortunately, vital records information specific to the Medicaid population is not available. This means, for example, that we can judge a newborn's condition at birth by hospitalization diagnoses and length of stay, but we cannot tell whether the baby lived.

Subject to the limitations of these data sources, this chapter asks five questions:

Screening
　　1. Were Medicaid pregnant women and infants screened?
　　2. What risk factors were found?
　　3. Were channeled women in fact at higher risk?

Channeling
　　4. Did channeled women deliver at higher level hospitals?

Outcomes
　　5. Did channeling improve outcomes?

SCREENING

The High Risk Channeling Project requires that pregnant women be risk-screened at the first prenatal visit, and that newborns be risk-screened at birth. For the screenings, physicians use forms that the state provides. The physician is supposed to mail a copy of the form to the Office of High Risk Care, and is then permitted to bill Medicaid for a screening fee, initially $10. The data we have on screenings is based on counts of screening forms reaching the Office of High Risk Care.

Table 12.1 shows the number of screening forms for pregnancies received and counted by the Office of High Risk Care, for selected periods since the High Risk Channeling Project began in April 1986. The total number of pregnancy-ending hospital claims is also shown for those periods. Pregnancy-ending hospitalizations totaled here are those in diagnosis-related groups 370 to 375 (deliveries), 378 (ectopic pregnancy), and 380 to 381 (abortions).

There are a number of problems with this comparison. It is not ideal to compare counts of screening forms received with counts of hospitalizations during the same time period, because of the lag between screening and delivery. The amount of the lag varies considerably, depending on when the woman first seeks prenatal care and when the physician sends in the completed form. No direct match between screening forms and claims is feasible for this period, because information from forms of non-high risk patients was not computerized. Since there was no definitive way to lag the data, Table 12.1 uses no lag. The number of screening forms is greater than the number of pregnancies because women whose risk statuses change are re-screened. Without computerization, one cannot determine how many such repeat screenings there are. The number of screenings exceeds the number of screening forms, if not all forms are mailed in or counted.

TABLE 12.1. Pregnancy Screenings and Pregnancy-Ending Hospitalizations, Selected Periods

	Screening forms received	Pregnancy-ending hospital claims	Screenings as percent of hospital claims
Apr.–Dec. 1986	5849	6856	85%
1987	7875	11601	68%
Aug.–Nov. 1988	4159	5404	77%
Dec. 1988–Mar. 1989	5672	5524	103%

The number of pregnancies is greater than the number of hospitalizations shown in the table. The table number does not include miscarriages at home or in connection with hospitalizations for other diagnoses. Because of these problems the comparisons in Table 12.1 must be considered only as broad indicators.

Table 12.1 indicates that at first the Project achieved a reasonably high rate of screening, with 85% as many forms as hospitalizations. In 1987, screening compliance apparently fell. Late 1988 to early 1989 data show a dramatic increase to virtually full compliance. This increase may reflect a combination of: a new system at the Office of High Risk Care for tabulating screening forms, an increase to $20 in the reimbursement for screening, and intensive educational efforts aimed at providers during 1988.

Table 12.2 shows the number of infant screening forms reaching the Office of High Risk Care for selected periods. Compliance with the infant screening requirement was low in the Project's first year, and remains no better than two-thirds up to the most recent data available. Infant screenings are supposed to be done in the hospital by the pediatrician at the time of birth. Though the number of locations is less for infants than for pregnant women (hospitals rather than physicians' offices), compliance with the infant screening requirement is much less. Anecdotal evidence is that hospital staffs resist having to handle yet another paper form. The number of newborn hospitalizations is about 3% more than the number of newborns, due to transfers. Correcting for this would affect the percentages in Table 12.2 only slightly. Securing compliance with infant screening is a continuing problem for the High Risk Channeling Project.

TABLE 12.2. Infant Screenings and Newborn Hospitalizations, Selected Periods

Period	Screening forms received	Newborn hospital claims	Screenings as percent of hospital claims
Apr.–Dec. 1986	2053	6502	32%
1987	6956	11670	60%
Aug.–Nov. 1988	3413	5717	60%
Dec. 1988–Mar. 1989	3641	5708	64%

RISKS

The screening forms list specific clinical risk factors in pregnant women and infants. The risk factor lists were developed in consultation with the South Carolina Medical Association. The presence of any one risk factor suffices to qualify the patient for channeling.

Table 12.3 lists the risk factors for pregnancies, in order of their prevalence in 1988. The most common risk factor was having had a low birthweight baby previously. This accounts for over one-third of channeled women. The second most common risk factor is "other" as specified by the physician. Note that behavioral concerns, such as substance abuse, are not on the risk factor list. Reporting these as high risk factors would be at the discretion of the physician.

TABLE 12.3. Risk Factors in High Risk Channeled Pregnancies, 1988 (1,065 Pregnancies)

Count	Risk factor
347	Previous infant < 2500g
206	Current pregnancy other
104	Diabetes Mellitus
96	Last pregnancy other
93	Hypertensive vascular disease
72	Fetal death (previous)
56	Premature labor
42	Neonatal death (previous)
42	Upper Renal Tract Disease
41	Multiple Gestation
29	Heart Disease
27	Congenital Anomaly
22	Pre-Eclampsia
20	RH Sensitization
19	Sickle Cell Anemia
18	Premature Ruptured Membranes
18	Incompetent Cervix
16	Three Consecutive Spontaneous Abortions
14	History of Incompetent Cervix
5	Placenta Previa
1	Eclampsia

Table 12.4 shows the risk factors for infants (1987 is used because 1988 data were less complete). Over half of the infants' risks are "other," including those requiring both Level II and Level III hospitalization. Designation of infants as high risk is even more discretionary than designation of pregnancies. This contributes to the geographic variation in Project participation, to be discussed.

RISK DESIGNATION AND OUTCOMES

Birth outcome data from the Medicaid bills can help evaluate whether the women who were chosen for channeling were in fact at higher risk than nonchanneled Medicaid women. Figure 12.1 shows the distribution of diagnosis-related groups (DRGs) of babies who could be matched to women channeled by the Project, in comparison with the DRG distribution of other babies.

TABLE 12.4. Risks Factors for High Risk Channeled Infants, 1987 (670 Infants)

Count	Risk factor
242	Other, Level II hospitalization
147	Ventilation or endotracheal CPAP
131	Other, Level III hospitalization
113	Weight 1500–2000g
111	Weight < 1500g
63	Cardiorespiratory problem
44	Uncomplicated sepsis/meningitis
42	Complicated sepsis or meningitis
41	Mild hypoglycemia
13	Major surgery
12	Congenital malformation
8	Major congenital malformation
5	Persistent seizures
4	Easily controlled seizures
3	Severe hypoglycemia
3	Nasal CPAP
2	Localized infection

FIGURE 12.1. Diagnosis-Related Group (DRG) Distributions of Newborns Matched and Not Matched to HRCP Channeled Women, 1988

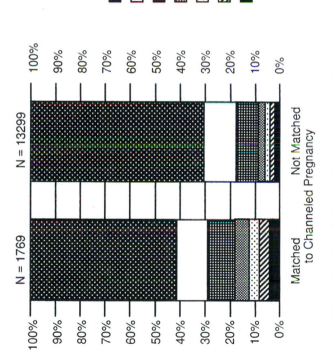

DRG

- 391 Normal Newborn
- 390 Full Other Prob
- 389 Full Major Prob
- 388 Premature
- 387 Prem Major Prob
- 386 Extreme Immature
- 385 Died or Transfer

N = 1769 N = 13299

Matched Not Matched
to Channeled Pregnancy

Source: University of South Carolina School of Public Health, 1988.

The matching was done by the Medicaid family number of the mother and infant, and by the dates of delivery and birth. From the database that the Department of Health and Environmental Control maintains on the Project participants, we extracted a list of individual Medicaid numbers of channeled women. These numbers were matched against Medicaid bills to find all deliveries to these women in 1988. The family Medicaid number and first day of hospital stay were taken from the hospital claim for each of these deliveries. These numbers and dates were then matched with newborn hospitalization claims, with the newborn considered to be the baby of a channeled mother if the Medicaid family numbers match and the hospitalization dates are within a month of each other. By this method, 1,769 infant claims for 1988 were matched to channeled mothers; 13,299 Medicaid newborns in 1988 were not matched.

There are some nonchanneled women in the same family with a channeled woman who happen to have a baby at about the same time as the channeled woman. These babies would be included in the matched group. This presumably tends to reduce the difference between the groups, so the actual difference in birth outcomes between channeled and nonchanneled mothers may be greater than what Figure 12.1 indicates.

Figure 12.1 shows that infants of channeled mothers are twice as likely to be premature as infants of nonchanneled Medicaid mothers. Nineteen percent of infants matched to channeled mothers are in the DRGs for died or transferred (385), extremely immature (386), or premature with and without major problems (387 and 388). Only 9.2% of nonmatched infants are in these DRGs. Among full-term infants (DRGs 390 and 391), the difference between the groups is less. 27% of the full-term newborns to channeled women had problems (DRG 390), compared with 23% for nonchanneled women.

The pattern shown in Figure 12.1 is confirmed by lengths of hospital stay. Babies of channeled mothers stayed an average of 5.43 days, compared with 3.74 days average for other Medicaid infants. There were 2.04 neonatal intensive care unit (NICU) days average per newborns of channeled mothers in 1988, more than double the 0.96 NICU days average per other Medicaid newborns.

Prematurity is evidently much more common among infants of channeled pregnancies than among other Medicaid infants. This should be taken as a positive, not a negative, reflection on the Project. Not even the best medical care can fully compensate for the pregnancy difficulties associated with clinical high risk conditions, such as diabetes and circulatory disease. Our findings confirm that the screening process has validity. Women selected for channeling do have a much higher likelihood of delivering infants who require extensive care.

CHANNELING AND DELIVERY HOSPITAL

The High Risk Channeling Project directs channeled women to deliver their babies at higher level hospitals. This is to make it more likely that complications of mother or baby can be treated on site without the risk and expense of transfer during a crisis. Claims data show that, statewide, 92.2% of channeled women delivered their babies at higher level hospitals in 1988, compared with 78.4% of nonchanneled Medicaid women.

The relative effect of the channeling policy is greatest among Medicaid women who live in counties that have only Level I hospitals. These women may incur significant travel costs, as well as red tape, to go out of county to a higher level hospital. Figure 12.2 shows that 85.5% of channeled women in these counties crossed a county line to deliver at a higher level hospital, compared with 60.2% of nonchanneled Medicaid women. Half of channeled women from these counties delivered at a Level III hospital, compared with 21.4% of nonchanneled Medicaid women. The breaking of barriers to access to higher level care for rural Medicaid patients may well be the Project's most important contribution.

OUTCOMES

Two standard ways of evaluating programs' outcomes are the case-control comparison and the before-after comparison. For the High Risk Channeling Project, no formal case-control comparison is possible because the Project was implemented statewide. No control areas were set aside so that outcomes without the Project could be compared to outcomes with the Project. The before-after method is

FIGURE 12.2. Level of Hospital of Delivery of Channeled and Nonchanneled Medicaid Women, Residents of Counties with Only Level I Hospitals, 1988

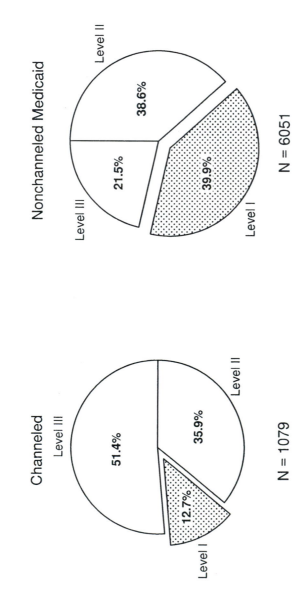

Channeled

Level III

51.4%

Level I

12.7%

Level II

35.9%

N = 1079

Nonchanneled Medicaid

Level II

38.6%

Level III

21.5%

Level I

39.9%

N = 6051

Source: University of South Carolina School of Public Health, 1988.

also not usable because, by coincidence, South Carolina Medicaid implemented prospective payment by diagnosis-related group (DRG) just before the Project began. The DRG-based payment system induced a jump in the newborn DRG distribution that swamped any possible effect of the Project. The proportion of newborn claims with prematurity or complications coded nearly tripled in just three months.

This chapter therefore explores two alternative approaches to outcome evaluation: a comparison of birth outcomes of high risk channeled women with outcomes of high risk women who were exempted from channeling; and a comparison of birth outcomes in counties identified as high, average, and low participants in the Project.

Exempts

The Project has, from its inception, allowed high risk women and parents of high risk infants to apply for exemptions from channeling. Possible reasons for exemptions include preferring one's own physician, lack of transportation to the high risk clinic, or lack of child care coverage during visits to the high risk clinic. Exemptions are granted at the discretion of the Office of High Risk Care, but in practice they were freely granted during the early years of the Project.

Exempts are self-selected controls. They have been judged high risk, like the channeled women, but they do not receive Project services. One might presume that women selecting themselves for exemption would tend to have less severe risks than those who go along with channeling to the high risk clinic. This would mean that a comparison of channeled women and exempts would tend to favor the exempts, if the Project services were no better than those available without the Project.

Figure 12.3 compares the DRG distribution in 1987 for infants matched (by Medicaid family number and date) to channeled women, exempt women, and other Medicaid women. Exempts had a worse birth outcome distribution than channeled women. Because of the relatively small number of exempts, this difference is statistically significant only at the 10% level. Both exempt and channeled women had worse birth outcomes than non-high risk women.

Table 12.5 shows that in 1987 the average length of stay for newborns of exempt women were slightly longer than for channeled women. The average number of neonatal intensive care unit

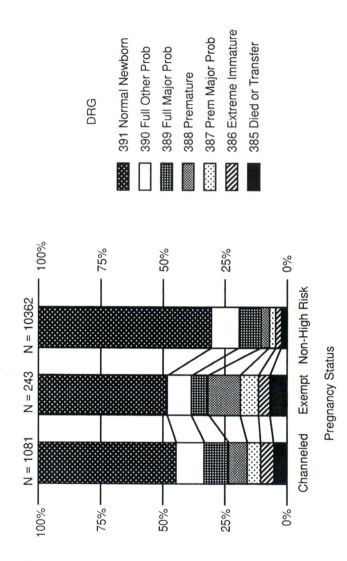

FIGURE 12.3. Birth Outcomes of Channeled, Exempt, and Non-High Risk Medicaid Pregnancies, 1987

DRG

391 Normal Newborn
390 Full Other Prob
389 Full Major Prob
388 Premature
387 Prem Major Prob
386 Extreme Immature
385 Died or Transfer

Pregnancy Status

Channeled   Exempt   Non-High Risk

Source: University of South Carolina School of Public Health, 1988.

TABLE 12.5. Average Length of Stay (LOS) and Average Neonatal Intensive Care Unit (NICU) Days per Newborn Hospitalization, by HRCP Status of Newborn's Mother*

	LOS	NICU days	Number of Hospital Claims
Exempt	6.68 (15.30)	2.98 (10.67)	243
Channeled	6.50 (15.62)	2.28 (9.58)	1081
Non-High Risk	4.27 (9.86)	1.20 (7.05)	10362

* Standard deviations in parentheses.

(NICU) days per newborn hospitalization was also higher for newborns of exempt women than channeled women. These differences are not statistically significant, but they do corroborate the finding in Figure 12.3 that exempts had worse outcomes than channeled women in 1987.

Figure 12.4 makes the same comparison for 1988. The picture changes. In 1988, the DRG distribution for newborns matched to exempt women was better than for newborns of channeled women, though still worse than the distribution for non-high risk Medicaid women. Confirming the change, Table 12.6 shows that in 1988 the average length of stay for newborns to exempt women was much less than for channeled women, and was actually slightly less than the average length of stay of newborns non-high risk women. The comparatively low standard deviation of length of stay for babies of exempt women indicates a relative absence of very long stays among newborns of these women.

Why the difference? The Office of High Risk Care had reported to us that in 1988, it improved its transportation capabilities and tightened its criteria for exemptions. The proportion of high risk women who were exempted fell from 18% in 1987 to 13% in 1988. The relatively smaller number of women exempted in 1988 were more likely to have been selected for having lower risk than the typical channeled woman. The tighter control on the pregnant women allowed to be exempted created a much lower risk popula-

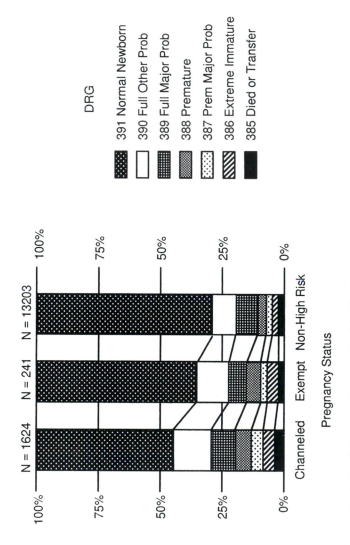

FIGURE 12.4. Comparison of Birth Outcomes: Channeled, Exempt, and Other Medicaid Pregnancies, 1988

Source: University of South Carolina School of Public Health.

TABLE 12.6. Average Length of Stay (LOS) and Average Neonatal Intensive Care Unit (NICU) Days per Newborn Hospitalization, by HRCP Status of Newborn's Mother*

	LOS	NICU days	Number of Hospital Claims
Exempt	3.60 (4.27)	0.77 (3.45)	241
Channeled	5.64 (11.98)	2.15 (9.05)	1,624
Not High Risk	3.74 (7.71)	0.96 (5.67)	13,203

* Standard deviations in parentheses.

tion in the exempted group, whose birth outcomes approximated those in the non-high risk group.

Thus, the 1987 data suggest that the Project was beneficial for high risk pregnancies. The 1988 data indicate that the better the Office of High Risk Care succeeds at reducing the demand for exemptions, the more biased a control group the exempts become.

County Comparison

Our second evaluation method is to compare birth outcomes across counties according to their Project participation. County participation is judged by the number of channeled pregnant women in the county. This number is compared with the number of channeled pregnant women that there would have been if the ratio of channeled pregnancies to all Medicaid pregnancies was the same as the statewide average. For example, Abbeville had 100 Medicaid-paid pregnancies in 1988. Statewide, 16.6% of deliveries were to channeled women, so the expected number of deliveries to channeled women from Abbeville was 16.6. The actual number was 19, so Abbeville was above average. To determine which counties were significantly different from average, the ratio of actual channeled to expected (in Abbeville's case, $19 \div 16.6 = 1.145$) is treated as the ratio of a Poisson variable to its expectation. The test for the significance of the ratio is described by Bailar and Ederer (1964).

Table 12.7 shows the calculation for all 46 counties of South Carolina. If the actual-to-expected ratio is significantly higher or

TABLE 12.7. County Variations in High Risk Channeled Deliveries, 1988

County	All Deliveries	Channeled Deliveries	Expected Channeled	Actual ÷ Expected Channeled	Ratio's Significance
Abbeville	100	19	16.6	1.145	
Aiken	377	55	62.6	0.879	
Allendale	119	32	19.7	1.620	High 5%
Anderson	434	57	72.0	0.791	
Bamberg	98	46	16.3	2.828	High 1%
Barnwell	176	45	29.2	1.541	High 1%
Beaufort	333	56	55.3	1.013	
Berkeley	328	58	54.4	1.066	
Calhoun	65	10	10.8	0.927	
Charleston	1350	172	224.0	0.768	Low 1%
Cherokee	211	23	35.0	0.657	Low 5%
Chester	204	23	33.9	0.679	
Chesterfield	215	31	35.7	0.869	
Clarendon	237	26	39.3	0.661	Low 5%
Colleton	237	39	39.3	0.992	
Darlington	403	46	66.9	0.688	Low 1%
Dillon	278	54	46.1	1.171	
Dorchester	238	55	39.5	1.393	High 1%
Edgefield	88	19	14.6	1.301	
Fairfield	125	19	20.7	0.916	
Florence	768	192	127.4	1.506	High 1%
Georgetown	285	48	47.3	1.015	
Greenville	959	142	159.1	0.892	
Greenwood	277	31	46.0	0.674	Low 5%
Hampton	158	17	26.2	0.648	
Horry	705	127	117.0	1.086	
Jasper	110	23	18.3	1.260	

TABLE 12.7 (continued)

Kershaw	191	38	31.7	1.199	
Lancaster	305	50	50.6	0.988	
Laurens	258	41	42.8	0.958	
Lee	158	48	26.2	1.831	High 1%
Lexington	344	49	57.1	0.858	
McCormick	30	4	5.0	0.803	
Marion	250	40	41.5	0.964	
Marlboro	200	24	33.2	0.723	
Newberry	154	27	25.6	1.056	
Oconee	138	18	22.9	0.786	
Orangeburg	572	153	94.9	1.612	High 1%
Pickens	258	45	42.8	1.051	
Richland	915	119	151.8	0.784	Low 5%
Saluda	85	15	14.1	1.063	
Spartanburg	693	96	115.0	0.835	
Sumter	562	101	93.3	1.083	
Union	122	23	20.2	1.136	
Williamsburg	265	44	44.0	1.001	
York	500	69	83.0	0.832	
TOTAL	14878	2469			

lower than 1 at the 5% or 1% significance level, a phrase indicating that appears in the Ratio's Significance column.

The Bailar and Ederer method takes into account that small counties tend to have more relative variation than large counties. The ratio required to be considered significant is further from 1 for a county with a few channeled deliveries than for a county with many channeled deliveries. For example, Chester, with an actual to expected ratio of 0.679, is not considered a significant outlier, while Darlington, with a ratio of 0.688, is. Darlington had twice the number of Medicaid deliveries as Chester in 1988, so its significance cutoff is closer to 1.

Among the 46 counties, one would expect 2.3 counties to be outliers at the 5% significance level simply by random variation, because 2.3 equals 5% of 46. One would expect 0.46 counties to be significant outliers at the 1% level. The fact that five counties are high outliers and two counties are low outliers at the 1% level means that the observed variation is greater than would be expected from purely random behavior. These counties are evidently doing something different, either positively or negatively. On the other hand, chance may be important in the cases of the two 5% high outliers and the four 5% low outliers.

In 1988, according to Table 12.7, Bamberg, Barnwell, Florence, Lee, and Orangeburg had significantly, at the 1% level, more channeled pregnancies than what would be expected from the statewide average rate. Allendale and Dorchester were higher than average at the 5% significance level. Charleston and Darlington had significantly low numbers of channeled pregnancies at the 1% level. Cherokee, Clarendon, Greenwood, and Richland were low at the 5% level.

To test for an outcome effect of the Project, counties with significantly few channeled women at the 5% level are considered low participators. Counties with significantly many channeled women at the 5% level are considered high participators.

Figure 12.5 shows that the newborn DRG distribution in the low participation counties as a group was worse than the DRG distributions for the other counties. A Chi-Square test shows the difference to be statistically significant at the .005 level. Of the newborn claims for residents of the low participation counties, 41.7% are in DRGs representing problems, compared with 29.4% with problems in the average participation counties and 28.6% in the high participation counties. Of the newborns from low participation counties, 2.7% were in DRG 386, the most severe for newborns, compared with 2.2% in the average counties and 2.1% in the high participation counties. The low participation counties had a much higher rate of complications among full-term babies. The DRG distributions of the high and average participation counties were almost identical.

An oddity, shown in Figure 12.5 is that the low participation counties has a lower frequency of DRG 385, which is for babies that died within two days or were transferred. This would seem contrary to the High Risk Channeling Project's goal of reducing the

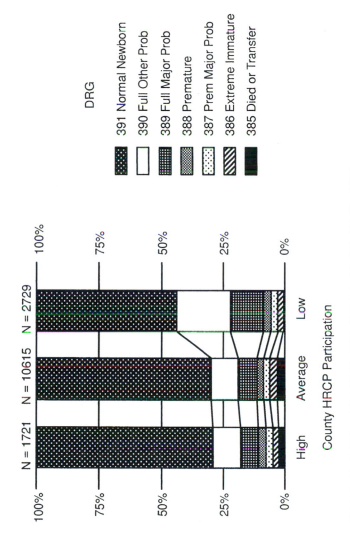

FIGURE 12.5. DRG Distributions of Newborns by County HRCP Participation, 1988

DRG

391 Normal Newborn
390 Full Other Prob
389 Full Major Prob
388 Premature
387 Prem Major Prob
386 Extreme Immature
385 Died or Transfer

County HRCP Participation

Source: University of South Carolina School of Public Health, 1988.

necessity for transfers. The explanation is that the low participation group is numerically dominated by two counties, Charleston and Richland, that have regional referral centers. The average and high participation groups also have regional referral centers among them, Greenville and Spartanburg for the average counties, and Florence for the high participation counties. In the low participation county group, however, the counties with tertiary centers account for a higher proportion of the births. Newborn residents of low participation counties who have problems are likely to have been born at the referral center, and thus not require transfer. A problem baby born in one of the average or high participation counties is more likely to require transfer, because the baby was less likely to have been born at a referral center in the first place.

This raises the question of whether the worse outcomes in the low participation counties is attributable to the predominance of the referral centers. The answer is that the DRG distributions in Figure 12.5 are by county of residence of the newborn, not by location of the hospital. For example, if a woman resident of Dorchester county delivers her baby at a hospital in Charleston, her baby's claim is counted with the high participation group, which Dorchester is in, and not the low participation group, which Charleston is in. The presence of a regional referral center in the county should not affect the DRG distribution of newborns to county residents.

The county comparison, like the exempt-channeled comparison, is subject to biased self-selection. Providers in the low participation counties selected themselves, in effect, for inclusion in that group. It may be that other characteristics of these counties are causing both their low participation in the Project and their elevated rates of problem newborns.

CONCLUSION

The South Carolina High Risk Channeling Project has had an impact on the poor's access to medical services for pregnant women. The most recent data indicate virtually complete high risk screenings. Channeled women generally do deliver their babies at higher level hospitals. Comparisons of birth outcomes of exempt versus channeled women and across counties that participate in the Project to different degrees indicate a birth outcome improvement associated with the Project, but these comparisons may be subject to selection bias.

During the period of the High Risk Channeling Project, South Carolina expanded Medicaid eligibility to all pregnant women and infants with family incomes up to 185% of the federal poverty level. This includes 40% of the state's births. For this expanded population, the state is building on the High Risk Channeling Project to provide a range of appropriate risk-graded care to all lower-income women and infants. No longer a program just for the poorest of the poor, Medicaid has become a major force in obstetric care, and is using its position to expand access to services that promise to reduce infant mortality and morbidity.

REFERENCE

Bailar JC, and Ederer F. Significance Factors for the Ratio of a Poisson Variable to its Expectation. *Biometrics* 1964; 639–643.

Chapter 13

American Indian Uranium Millworkers: A Study of the Perceived Effects of Occupational Exposure

Susan E. Dawson
Gary E. Madsen

BACKGROUND

The uranium boom on the Colorado Plateau (an area including the states of Arizona, Colorado, New Mexico, and Utah) occurred from the late 1940s through the 1960s. During this period, thousands of uranium mines and 23 processing mills were built to supply the United States government with uranium for the growing atomic energy program. Hundreds of these mines were developed on the Navajo Reservation along with four uranium processing mills. It has been estimated that, working both on and off the reservation, approximately 3,000 Navajo worked in the mines and about 1,000 worked in the mills.

The association between underground uranium mining and disease has been well documented in epidemiologic studies (Archer, 1983; Gottlieb and Husen, 1982; Samet et al., 1984b). Among the illnesses identified were lung cancer and respiratory diseases, specifically, pulmonary fibrosis, silicosis, and pneumoconiosis which

This chapter was originally published in *Journal of Health & Social Policy*, Vol. 7(2) 1995.

The authors would like to thank the College of Humanities, Arts, and Social Sciences of Utah State University for travel support. They would also like to thank Victor E. Archer, MD, and David Drown, PhD, for helpful comments concerning the study.

are caused primarily by exposure to radon and its progeny and silica dust. In 1990, in response to these studies and public pressure, Congress enacted the Radiation Exposure Compensation Act (RECA), providing compassionate payment to underground uranium miners and certain other groups exposed to radiation.

Epidemiologic studies identifying illnesses related to uranium milling are not as conclusive as the mining studies, and the millers have not been included in RECA. The most comprehensive studies to date are of Anglo uranium millworkers. These were conducted by Archer, Wagoner, and Lundin (1973) and by Waxweiler et al. (1983). In neither study were excess rates of lung cancer indicated. Archer, Wagoner, and Lundin (1973) did find a statistically significant excess of malignant disease of lymphatic and hematopoietic tissue, and Waxweiler et al. (1983) found a statistically significant excess of nonmalignant respiratory disease (NMRD) which includes emphysema, fibrosis, silicosis, and chronic obstructive pulmonary disease. As a distinct group, the American Indian uranium millworkers have never been studied. Wagoner et al. (1964) studied American Indian workers but did not differentiate the millers from the miller/miners.

Traditionally, researchers who study uranium occupational exposure have relied upon methods relating occupational exposure with physical disease outcomes using objective indices. For example, dust and radiation levels are monitored in work areas, and these levels are then related to possible occupational disease outcomes. It has been pointed out by Roberts (1993), however, that there is also a need to study the social/psychological impacts of exposure to technological events. He notes that people's perceptions of exposure can be related to feelings of stress which can trigger psychological effects, e.g., depression and anxiety. Fenton (1993), who has studied the importance of emotional and perceptual aspects of health and illness, also supports this view of the important connection between the mind and body. In this study, we examined the interconnections of people's perceptions of workplace hazard exposures and physical and emotional health.

SAMPLE AND METHOD

A case study of 81 American Indian uranium millworkers was conducted by the authors in the Fall of 1992 on the Navajo Reservation in Shiprock, New Mexico, and Tonalea, Arizona. It was not intended to be an epidemiologic study, but rather exploratory in nature, concentrating on identifiable cases. Initially, the stimulus for this study began when one of the authors was approached by several millers at a Senate field hearing in Shiprock in 1990. The workers requested that a study of their group be undertaken to document their work histories.

The sample included 78 Navajo men and three Hopi women. All the respondents worked in the mills during the 1950s and 1960s, with only one worker employed after 1970. The sample contained 68 (84.0%) former millers and 13 (16.0%) widows of deceased millers. Millers were included in the study if they had worked at least one year in uranium milling. Seventy-five worked at one mill, five at two mills, and one at three mills. Seven mills, on and off the reservation, were represented in the sample, but over 80% were employed at only two of the seven mills.

Obtaining a sample of American Indian uranium millers, let alone a representative sample, was a difficult task. We were informed by milling company representatives that, prior to 1970, company personnel records did not identify ethnic/racial data on employees. These records contained only names and addresses. The addresses, however, were often listed as "General Delivery" or general locations, such as living in or near Shiprock. Because of confidentiality, we were unable to secure a list from the Office of Navajo Uranium Workers, a registry that includes about 150 Navajo uranium millers.

The sample was gathered using a combination of techniques. News releases in local newspapers and public announcements on local radio stations were directed at possible respondents. In addition, key informants who knew millers were asked to notify them of the study. Certain chapter houses on the Navajo Reservation were designated as interview venues. Key informants were also asked to identify the names and possible locations of millers they knew so that additional contacts could be made personally at their residences. Once interviews began, each respondent was asked for the names and possible locations of any other millers who could be contacted. About half the respondents were interviewed in the chapter houses and the other half at the respondents' residences.

The data were gathered through in-depth interviews. Major content areas included personal descriptive information about each respondent, an occupational history, the respondents' perceptions of working conditions at the uranium mill(s), and a health history. The widows were asked the above information regarding their husbands. Because the authors did not have access to medical records, the health histories were largely self-reported. In some cases, respondents produced a portion of their medical records, but this generally was not the rule.

Unlike a previous study of Navajo uranium miners (Dawson, 1992), interpreters were generally not needed because most respondents spoke English. A former mill manager explained that workers needed to understand and speak English in order to work in the mills. Since American Indian and Anglo workers were in a highly integrated workplace, they needed to coordinate activities around the work process.

The median age of the millers interviewed was 60, ranging from 78 to 46 years of age. The highest level of formal education was four years of college and the lowest was no formal education. The median level of education was eight years.

FINDINGS

Working Conditions

Uranium milling involves crushing and leaching the extracted ore and drying it in furnaces to obtain U_3O_8, a concentrate of uranium oxides more commonly known as yellowcake. Some mills also processed vanadium as well as uranium. According to Archer (1981), Beverly (1960), and Miller, Holaday, and Doyle (1956), radon daughters were perceived as posing little threat in uranium mills because of the open construction of the buildings. The greatest hazards were considered to be airborne radioactive materials such as uranium, thorium, and radium (Archer, 1981). Other hazards include airborne silica, vanadium (where processed), acids, and alkalis. Also, radium may produce high gamma radiation in areas where there is accumulation on equipment (Archer et al., 1962).

Each respondent was asked to supply a comprehensive work history. All had worked at least one year in uranium milling. Of the 81 millers, 53 (65.4%) had been uranium millers only, and 28 (34.6%) had been both millers and miners. The number of years worked in uranium mills ranged from one to 14, with a median of six years.

How did the respondents perceive the work environment? They were asked to describe the working conditions at each uranium mill in which they worked. Since some workers were employed in more than one mill, this resulted in 81 respondents being asked to provide 88 descriptions. Three respondents did not provide descriptions, leaving 78 respondents providing 85 descriptions of mills. A content analysis of this question yielded two predominant workplace hazards: dust and fumes in the mill(s). Sixty-four (75.3%) of the 85 descriptions mentioned one or both of these environmental factors. The dusty conditions were identified with front-end operations involving the ore such as unloading, weighing, crushing, conveying, and sampling, as well as end-product operations involving yellowcake and vanadium barreling. Fumes were mentioned by those who worked in the leaching process where caustic chemicals such as sulfuric acid were used. In addition, the respondents identified uranium and vanadium fumes emitted by the fusion furnaces.

The former millers in this sample were asked to identify any personal protective equipment used in performance of their work. The items most often mentioned were respirators and gloves, which were worn by a majority of the respondents; however, many unsolicited comments were made concerning the respirators. Among them were problems related to the sporadic availability of replacement filters and respirators during their employment. In addition, some workers said that the wearing of respirators was not required, and they did not always wear them. Moreover, most of these workers reported that they were not informed of the hazards of radiation, and therefore were unlikely to take extra precautions to protect themselves.

Examples of mill environment descriptions by the respondents are as follows:

> It wasn't clean. It was too dusty and you had to eat right at the mill. It was noisy. We had respirators but they really didn't work. The ore dust is really fine stuff, and the respirators didn't stop it.

I worked both sides of the ovens that dried yellowcake and vanadium. Mostly worked in the vanadium side. I worked at the mill for ten years. The first time I worked, I thought it was clean. The vanadium side was hot steam. There was a lot of dust when we were packing in both sides. But I wanted a job.

It was messy and disorganized. It was also very dusty. I had an instant headache while working there. Also much coughing. In the first four years, they didn't provide masks. I breathed much dust and even coughed up the dust. I also had it in my eyes, and it irritated my eyes. I also had sores on my feet. It was hot and I had to wear an acid protector suit. Yellowcake would get into the suit.

The whole building was enclosed. Very stuffy. Can smell the boiling acid and ammonia. We had to handle this stuff (yellowcake) with our bare hands. When I worked in the yellowcake, I only wore a respirator. The dust was there all the time, especially when the yellowcake was being barreled. Now I see those who work in the nuclear area wear special clothing, but we didn't.

The dust and fume hazards these millers experienced were also noted by United States Public Health Service (USPHS) personnel who discussed health protection of uranium millers in the mid-1950s (Miller et al., 1956). Control of dust arising from ore crushing ranged from fair to poor. It was further noted that, "Relatively high concentrations of uranium and vanadium fumes were found around the fusion furnaces" (Miller, Holaday, and Doyle, 1956:54).

Duncan Holaday, who as a USPHS industrial hygienist inspected mills during the early period of uranium production, noted that one of the mills on the Navajo Reservation was "a real mess" in relation to cleanliness (Ambler, 1980:4). Referring to mills in general, he also stated that mill operators did try to uphold hygiene standards; however, the mill managers' attempts were often unproductive. For example, Holaday stated, "They put in fancy ventilators that just got all the dust circulating, because they hadn't bothered to clean up first" (Ambler, 1980:4). In addition, several mill managers who were interviewed by the authors indicated that during the period of the 1950s and 1960s the mills' emphasis on health and safety varied.

HEALTH PROBLEMS

Physical Health

Millworkers provided medical histories as part of the interview process. Respondents either knew a medical diagnosis or they were only able to describe symptoms. A wide array of health problems were reported including: problems relating to cardiovascular, respiratory, and renal systems; eye problems; and cancer, rashes, and arthritis. Only four respondents indicated no illnesses or illness symptoms.

We will limit ourselves to a discussion of cancer, respiratory problems, and rashes. Certain cancer and respiratory problems have been identified previously in the studies of uranium millers and miners. Rashes, however, have not been identified in the literature but were often identified in this study. Two controls were also introduced. The first control variable included separating those respondents who were millers from those who were uranium miners and millers. In this way, the possible effects of uranium mining could be assessed since the health problems of miners are well documented. The second control variable was cigarette smoking behavior which was introduced when looking at respiratory problems.

There were seven (8.6%) cases of cancer identified by the 81 respondents. Three cases were reported among millers and four among miller/miners. Cancer cases included one with prostate, two with stomach, one with thyroid, and three with unknown types of cancer. Of this "Unknown" category, one respondent reported possible bladder cancer and one suggested cancer of the leg. There were no reported cases of lung cancer, as there had been with the miners, or lymphatic cancer and hematopoietic cancer which have been found among Anglo millworkers.

Respiratory problems were among the most often reported types of health problems. Sixty (74.1%) of the respondents reported one or more respiratory problems, including bronchitis, pneumonia, tuberculosis, and lung congestion. Frequent colds, persistent coughs, and shortness of breath were the three most identified symptoms. Frequent colds were reported by 25 (30.9%) of the respondents. Thirty-five (43.2%) of the respondents reported that they had persistent coughs, and 26 (32.1%) identified shortness of breath. We analyzed persistent coughs and shortness of breath in more detail since they had been studied previously among uranium miners.

Because respiratory problems can be caused by cigarette smoking, cigarette smoking behavior was important to document. Four smoking categories were developed based upon the respondents' reported cigarette smoking behaviors: individuals who had never smoked; light smokers (three or fewer cigarettes per day); moderate smokers (four to 19 cigarettes per day); and heavy smokers (20 cigarettes or more per day). Furthermore, categories identified as "past" were created because many had quit smoking, most of them 20 or more years ago. Fifty-five percent of the sample never smoked, and three-quarters were either nonsmokers or light smokers who had quit 20 or more years ago. The low incidence of cigarette smoking of these workers is supported by past studies of smoking behavior among American Indian workers (Archer, Gillam, and Wagoner, 1976; Samet et al., 1984a; Sievers, 1968).

Tables 13.1 and 13.2 present findings concerning persistent cough and shortness of breath, controlling for cigarette smoking behavior and for employment as millers or miller/miners. Twenty-four (45.3%) of the millers and 11 (39.3%) of the miller/miners reported persistent coughing. Sixteen (30.2%) of the millers and ten (35.7%) of the miller/miners reported shortness of breath. Over 70% of both the millers and miller/miners with persistent coughing or shortness of breath were nonsmokers or were light smokers many years ago.

Archer et al. (1964) conducted a morbidity study of uranium miners in 1957 and 1960. Amount of radiation exposure was related to several diseases and symptoms including persistent cough and shortness of breath. Since we gathered data on persistent cough and shortness of breath, a comparison can be made with this previous work. Archer et al. (1964) found that 27% of the miners with high radiation exposure, who were heavy smokers and represented the oldest cohort (35 years and older), complained of persistent cough, and 21.4% indicated shortness of breath. For the same age cohort, who were nonsmokers and had low radiation exposure, the results were

TABLE 13.1. Persistent Cough and Cigarette Smoking

Persistent Cough

Cigarette Smoking Behavior	Millers		Miller/Miners		Total	
	N	%	N	%	N	%
Never smoked	12	52.2	4	40.0	16	48.5
Light smoker (past)	6	26.1	5	50.0	11	33.3
Light smoker (present)	2	8.7	1	10.0	3	9.1
Moderate smoker (past)	2	8.7	—	—	2	6.1
Heavy smoker (past)	1	4.3	—	—	1	3.0
Total	23	100.0	10	100.0	33	100.0

TABLE 13.2. Shortness of Breath and Smoking

Shortness of Breath

Cigarette Smoking Behavior	Millers		Miller/Miners		Total	
	N	%	N	%	N	%
Never smoked	9	64.3	5	62.5	14	63.6
Light smoker (past)	1	7.1	1	12.5	2	9.1
Light smoker (present)	1	7.1	2	25.0	3	13.6
Heavy smoker (past)	1	7.1	—	—	1	4.5
Heavy smoker (present)	1	7.1	—	—	1	4.5
Other	1	7.1	—	—	1	4.5
Total	14	100.0	8	100.0	22	100.0

5.3% for persistent cough and 2.8% for shortness of breath. In the present study all respondents were 46 years of age and older, and the largest category of smoking behavior consisted of individuals who had never smoked. Of the 30 nonsmoking millers, 12 (40.0%) indicated persistent cough and nine (30.0%) identified shortness of breath. Corresponding results for the 15 nonsmoking miller/miners were five

(33.3%) with persistent cough and four (26.7%) with shortness of breath. One must be cautious in making a comparison between the present study and Archer's study of uranium miners. For one thing, the millers in this study are an older cohort and might be expected to have higher rates of these respiratory problems coincident to age. However, shortness of breath and chronic cough could be symptomatic of more serious pulmonary problems.

Chronic obstructive pulmonary disease, emphysema, pulmonary fibrosis, scarred lungs, and silicosis were also reported by some of the respondents. These illnesses have been previously identified among Anglo uranium millers (Waxweiler et al., 1983). Out of the 81 respondents, there were eight (9.9%) reported cases of these problems; half of these cases occurred among millers and the other half among miller/miners. There were only two smoking groups represented, individuals who had never smoked and those who had smoked lightly in the past. All of the miller/miners had never smoked. Of that group, one had chronic obstructive pulmonary disease, one had scarred lungs, and two had silicosis. Of the miller group, only one had smoked lightly in the past and he had pulmonary fibrosis. In the never smoked category, there was one miller with emphysema and two millers with scarred lungs. The workers who reported these respiratory illnesses had been diagnosed by physicians.

A high occurrence of rashes also was found among the uranium millworkers. Forty-eight (59.3%) reported having rashes, with 32 (60.4%) in the millers' group and 16 (57.1%) in the miller/miners' group. Twenty-seven (56.3%) of the 48 stated that their rashes began during or after their work at the mills. In addition to rashes, three of the respondents (3.7%) reported "rotting toenails" in which the toenails became soft, fell off, and were difficult to regrow.

These results show similar reports of respiratory problems and rashes between the millers and the miller/miners, and they do not suggest that smoking is an important contributor to the respiratory problems. It is therefore possible that such problems are related to the millwork, given the employees' exposures to dust and chemicals.

We felt it was also important to understand whether the millworkers perceived any of their illnesses/symptoms to be work-related. Respondents were asked if they believed they had a health problem(s) related to their millwork. Sixty (74.1%) of the 81 answered yes, 11 (13.6%) answered no, and ten (12.3%) said that they were unsure.

Emotional Health

Respondents were asked if they had any health problems which affected them emotionally. Twenty-eight (34.6%) of the 81 respondents expressed anxiety related to their health problems, and 23 (28.4%) of the respondents experienced depression. In all, 39 (48.1%) of the 81 respondents experienced anxiety, depression, or both. In addition to anxiety and depression related to their own health, 29 of the respondents indicated concern about other millworkers' deaths, and eight indicated concern about other millworkers' sicknesses.

The following comments are examples of respondents' reported anxiety and depression. One widow described her husband's emotional state when he was alive: "A few years later all the people he worked with passed away. His mind passed from positive to negative." Another respondent was under a psychiatrist's care for chronic depression at the time of the interview. Speaking for him throughout the interview, his wife stated that he blames the company for his emotional problem. She also indicated that he worries constantly about what may happen to him and his family because of his work at the mill. Other emotional problems identified by some respondents included "weakness," loneliness, frustration, not feeling well, not sleeping well, not eating well, grief, confused thoughts, sadness, and withdrawal from family and friends.

Concern about future health problems developing, e.g., birth defects, was also expressed. A former miller reported her views about the cause of her child's birth defect:

> It was interpreted to me at the time I had my deformed baby that this kind of work was not good in terms for the people of the universe. That [uranium] harms people. There we may get our after effects later on in the years that come. So I always kind of expect these illnesses would come.

In addition, several workers appeared to have a fatalistic view about their health. A spouse noted that her husband "knows what's going to kill him and it's the uranium." The feeling of contracting an inevitable illness from the uranium was expressed by several respondents. As a concerned worker noted, "One person who worked there and has died said you get sick 15 to 30 years later. It takes time." Respondents also expressed concern about other workers' sicknesses or their illnesses. One former miller stated, "It bothers me emotionally to see other workers sick and worse off than I am. That's why I'm involved with the former millworkers [support group]. . . . We want to see these people with us a little more longer."

It has been reported previously that 60 (74.1%) of the 81 respondents believed they had a health problem(s) related to their millwork. This was then compared with reported anxiety and depression. We found that of the 21 respondents who answered either "no" or "unsure" as to whether their health problem(s) were work-related, only three (14.3%) reported anxiety, depression, or both. However, of the 60 who felt they had a health problem(s) related to their millwork, 36 (60.0%) reported experiencing anxiety, depression, or both. Several respondents expressed considerable anxiety and concern throughout the interviews regarding their health status and occupational exposure.

Workers and workers' widows explained that they were worried about health problems related to the uranium process both for themselves and their families. A widow of a worker explained, "He [her husband] knew he would die when he coughed. [He said], 'I'll be the next one.' Several men died. . . . Here we thought the uranium made us money, and now here we are sick." One respondent stated, "Now I worry that my health problems are because of my work at the mill." Another said, "I think [the] mill job is catching up with me. It all depends on the man upstairs if I get sicker."

In addition, lack of understanding about health professionals' diagnoses elicited concern and anxiety. One respondent, who was told there was nothing wrong with him, disagreed saying, "They say there is nothing wrong, but I think there is something wrong." Another respondent stated, "When I was working at the mill, I developed a growth on the forehead. It was like a root. I went to the hospital . . . and I had it removed by a doctor. The doctor wasn't too sure it was related to the mill job, but he thought it might be."

SUMMARY AND DISCUSSION

This study of American Indian uranium millworkers was exploratory in nature regarding some of the possible effects of uranium milling. The results indicate that the workers had vivid recollections of the dust and fume hazards associated with the work environment, even though more than 20 years had passed since their mill employment. Many health problems were reported by the respondents. Two of the most frequently identified were respiratory problems and rashes. Whether or not any of these or others are caused by uranium millwork has yet to be determined, but it is important to recognize that a majority of the respondents felt they had health problem(s) related to their millwork. A previous study by Waxweiler et al. (1983) has already identified respiratory problems among Anglo workers. However, this category of illnesses needs to be further addressed among the American Indian population. As a health problem affecting uranium millworkers, the rash symptoms have not been identified previously in the literature and also need to be studied further.

In addition to reporting physical symptoms, many respondents said they were experiencing emotional problems related to their physical illnesses. Anxiety and depression concerning their health and the health of other miller friends were the most identified forms of stress. The people most likely to report emotional problems were those who felt their illnesses were the result of their millwork. As Thomas and Thomas pointed out many years ago, if people "define situations as being real, they are real in their consequences" (Thomas and Thomas, 1928:572). This points out the importance of Robert's (1993) recognition that perceived occupationally-related illness can result in psychological stress.

The problems experienced by these former uranium millworkers need to be addressed in a serious and timely fashion. The millworkers themselves have formed a grassroots support group in Shiprock called The Four Corners Navajo Uranium Millers Association. The group, which provides technical assistance and support to millers, is in the process of expanding across the reservation.

To address the concerns of these people, we feel a medical screening and full examination of patient medical records is needed, not only for those in this sample but for other former millers who might be experiencing similar problems. A screening would identify any illnesses among the millworkers' group. Health professionals, including nurses, physicians, and social workers, need to be aware of the problems associated with the millworkers and could work directly with them in the screening process and the support group. This could work toward alleviating stress among the workers who are not sure of the exact nature of their problems.

In addition, an epidemiologic study is necessary to establish any correlation between work exposure and occupational illness for the miller population. Given that the American Indian millworkers have not been studied, their inclusion in a retrospective epidemiologic study would provide a basis for policy-making decisions regarding their current physical and emotional health.

REFERENCES

Ambler, M. (1980). Ailing uranium millworkers seek recognition, aid. *High Country News, 12*(17), 1–4.

Archer, V.E. (1981). Health concerns in uranium mining and milling. *Journal of Occupational Medicine, 23*(7), 502.

Archer, V.E. (1983). Diseases of uranium miners. In Rom, W.M. (ed.), *Environmental and occupational medicine.* Boston: Little, Brown and Company, 687–691.

Archer, V.E., Carrol, B.E., Brinton, H.P., and Saccomanno, G. (1964). Epidemiological studies of some non-fatal effects of uranium mining. In Proceedings of a Symposium, Vienna 26–31, August 1963. *Radiological health and safety in mining and milling of nuclear materials, volume 1.* Jointly organized by IAEA, ILO, WHO: 21–35.

Archer, V.E., Gillam, J.D., and Wagoner, J.K. (1976). Respiratory disease mortality among uranium miners. *Annals of the New York Academy of Sciences, 271,* 280–293.

Archer, V.E., Magnuson, H.J., Holaday, D.A., and Lawrence, P.A. (1962). Hazards to health in uranium mining and milling. *Journal of Occupational Medicine, 4*(2), 55–60.

Archer, V.E., Wagoner, J.K., and Lundin, F.E. (1973). Cancer mortality among uranium mill workers. *Journal of Occupational Medicine, 15*(1), 11–14.

Beverly, R.G. (1960). Progress in radiation control in uranium mines and mills. Unpublished paper presented at the National Western Mining and Energy Conference. Denver, CO, 22 April 1960. Union Carbide Nuclear Co., Grand Junction, CO.

Dawson, S.E. (1992). Navajo uranium workers and the effects of occupational illnesses: A case study. *Human Organization: Journal of the Society for Applied Anthropology, 51*(4), 389–397.

Fenton, D. (1993). The brain and immune system. In Moyers, B. *Health and the mind,* 213–238. New York: Doubleday.

Gottlieb, L.S., and Husen, L.A. (1982). Lung cancer among Navajo uranium miners. *Chest, 81,* 449–452.

Miller, S.E., Holaday, D.A., and Doyle, H.N. (1956). Health protection of uranium miners and millers. *AMA Archives of Industrial Health, 14,* 48–55.

Roberts, J.T. (1993). Psychosocial effects of workplace hazardous exposures: Theoretical synthesis and preliminary findings. *Social Problems, 40*(1), 74–86.

Samet, J.M., Kutvirt, D.M., Waxweiler, R.J., and Key, C.R. (1984a). Uranium mining and lung cancer in Navajo men. *New England Journal of Medicine, 310*(23), 1481.

Samet, J.M., Young, R.A., Morgan, M.V., Humble, C.G., Epler, G.R., and McLoud, T.C. (1984b). Prevalence survey of respiratory abnormalities in New Mexico uranium miners. *Health Physics, 46*(2), 361–370.

Sievers, M.L. (1968). Cigarette and alcohol usage by southwestern American Indians. *American Journal of Public Health, 58,* 71–82.

Thomas, W.I., and Thomas, D. (1928). *The child in America.* New York: Alfred A. Knopf.

Wagoner, J.K., Archer, V.E., Carrol, B.E., Holaday, D.A., and Lawrence, P.A. (1964). Cancer mortality patterns among U.S. uranium miners and millers, 1950 through 1962. *Journal of the National Cancer Institute, 32*(4), 787–801.

Waxweiler, R.J., Archer, V.E., Roscoe, R.J., Watanabe, A., and Thun, M.J. (1983). Mortality patterns among a retrospective cohort of uranium mill workers. Proceedings of the Sixteenth Midyear Topical Meeting of the Health Physics Society, Inhalation Toxicology Research Institute, 428–435.

Epilogue

Health and Poverty:
Below the Bottom Line

Michael J. Holosko
Marvin D. Feit

This compilation of recent and topical empirical articles selected and edited from the *Journal of Health & Social Policy* exhibits our understanding of substantive issues related to health and poverty in North America and provides examples of their occurrence. They serve as testimony to the fact that there are endemic problems with our health care system that have severe consequences for individuals who are poor, e.g. higher incidence of disease and illness, greater mortality and morbidity, inferior health care practices, a lack of use or faith in the health care systems, social and psychologic sequelae, etc. However one views this issue—the picture is bleak.

Despite our bias for health care reform, we do not anticipate that the overall health of the poor will be significantly improved as a result of structural changes which may occur in the system. Indeed, not one of the issues presented in this text will be resolved should national health care, and/or universal coverage become a reality, unless it is accompanied by large-scale social, cultural, and value shifts in our thinking. Further, we contend that the economic disparity in American society will continue to undermine any attempts at achieving such "universality." In Kuhnian terms, a decided paradigm shift is required in order to effect such a change. One of the more intriguing questions is—can North American society adapt to accommodate an ideological shift in its thinking? Only time will tell.

Two endemic features of American society which have historically been seen as the most divisive issues in its evolution to date are socioeconomic status and race. These issues serve as the polarizing determinants which have been structurally ingrained into the existing medical and health care policies and programs as evidenced in this text. Figure 1 presents a conceptual matrix showing their interrelationship to one another, as well as their structural relationship to health care policies, and programs for poor people.

The demarcations in quadrant III indicate that if you are poor and in a minority group in this country, you are likely to be receiving no care or substandard health care and are clearly "below the line" and

FIGURE 1

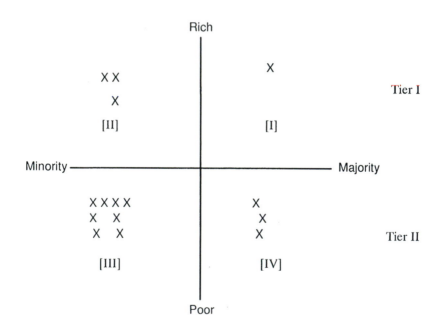

Note: X = Health care consequences: substandard care, no care, lack of access to care, unequal care, greater illness and disease, poor health care practices, higher incidence of morbidity and mortality, greater frequency of uninsured persons, more at-risk health behaviors, fewer prevention or health promotion activities, etc.

in Tier II. Quadrant III also depicts the greater frequency of resultant health care consequences, e.g. greater illness and disease, lack of access care, unequal care, higher morbity and mortality, etc., that occur to such individuals. Indeed, Section II of this book provides rich examples of individuals and programs in quadrant III.

Tier I represents persons who are "above the line" and in preferential health care situations in North America, usually demarked by their employment/insurance status. As a result, quadrants I and II may become indistinguishable along the x-axis of the majority-minority continuum. Lateral movement in Tier I (between quadrants I and II), and in Tier II (quadrants III and IV) typifies the best-case scenario for any resultant modification in the current health care system. This lateral movement is likely to occur regardless of any modification in health care restructuring or reform. Thus, some myths, such as better access equals better care, may be perpetrated by these lateral movements within the Tiers. For example, minority persons in Tier I are likely to face racial or cultural issues in their treatment or care despite having health care insurance.

In this matrix, quadrant I (rich and majority) holds the potential for individuals to receive the best health care and the ensuing benefits of the system on a regular basis. In quadrant I, there are sustaining mechanisms which have perpetrated the separation that exists among these individuals and those who find themselves in the other three quadrants (II, III and IV). Obvious examples include the historically powerful lobbying of the American Medical Association, the insurance industry, and other key health care providers who perpetuate divisiveness among the subgroups in this society; the lip service paid to prevention programs; the urbanization of health care; and the replacement of economic imperatives over cultural and individual medical and health care needs. Undermining these examples is a majority- and case-driven value system that perpetuates such divisiveness.

The matrix also reveals some interesting insights regarding the relationship between health and poverty. As indicated in this book, it becomes increasingly clear that a large portion of public policy emanates from the populations who find themselves in quadrant III—while the primary beneficiaries of these policies are located in quadrants I and II, or those with money. For instance, the chapters by McPhee, Nolan, and Dawson and Madsen provide examples of this relationship. As well, Dawson and Madsen note that American Indian uranium millworkers have been excluded from epidemiologic studies identifying illnesses related to uranium milling, and uranium millers have not been included in the Radiation Exposure Compensation Act of 1990. In this example, being classified as "poor" ostensively excluded the American Indian uranium millworkers from consideration for study and for any possible health benefits.

Several chapters were also included in this book as examples of programs considered successful or that made a contribution to the health care needs of the poor. In our view, these programs serve only to "bridge" the gap or "blur" the distinction between the populations located in quadrant IV (poor and deserving) and quadrant III (poor and undeserving). Such programs appear to enable certain select subgroups of poor people to be intermittently served by health care providers. Thus, high-risk pregnant mothers, young children from poor families, people with HIV/AIDS, and so forth are the recipients of research and demonstration or "pilot" programs, intended to move a select sample into receiving health care, while retaining their "poor" status. Such realities continue to perpetuate the existing divisiveness between Tiers I and II. Thus, the rich are seldom affected by or are exempt from participation in programs designed for the poor. In this way, the current two-tier health care system is maintained, while keeping alive the illusion of someday achieving universal coverage.

Index

Page numbers followed by the letter "t" indicate tables; those followed by the letter "f" indicate figures.

Order Your Own Copy of
This Important Book for Your Personal Library!

HEALTH AND POVERTY

_____in hardbound at $49.95 (ISBN: 0-7890-0149-7)

_____in softbound at $24.95 (ISBN: 0-7890-0228-0)

COST OF BOOKS_____

OUTSIDE USA/CANADA/
MEXICO: ADD 20%_____

POSTAGE & HANDLING_____
(US: $3.00 for first book & $1.25
for each additional book)
Outside US: $4.75 for first book
& $1.75 for each additional book)

SUBTOTAL_____

IN CANADA: ADD 7% GST_____

STATE TAX_____
(NY, OH & MN residents, please
add appropriate local sales tax)

FINAL TOTAL_____
(If paying in Canadian funds,
convert using the current
exchange rate. UNESCO
coupons welcome.)

☐ **BILL ME LATER:** ($5 service charge will be added)
(Bill-me option is good on US/Canada/Mexico orders only;
not good to jobbers, wholesalers, or subscription agencies.)

☐ Check here if billing address is different from
shipping address and attach purchase order and
billing address information.

Signature_____

☐ **PAYMENT ENCLOSED: $**_____

☐ **PLEASE CHARGE TO MY CREDIT CARD.**

☐ Visa ☐ MasterCard ☐ AmEx ☐ Discover
☐ Diner's Club

Account #_____

Exp. Date_____

Signature_____

Prices in US dollars and subject to change without notice.

NAME_____

INSTITUTION_____

ADDRESS_____

CITY_____

STATE/ZIP_____

COUNTRY_____ COUNTY (NY residents only)_____

TEL_____ FAX_____

E-MAIL_____
May we use your e-mail address for confirmations and other types of information? ☐ Yes ☐ No

Order From Your Local Bookstore or Directly From
The Haworth Press, Inc.
10 Alice Street, Binghamton, New York 13904-1580 • USA
TELEPHONE: 1-800-HAWORTH (1-800-429-6784) / Outside US/Canada: (607) 722-5857
FAX: 1-800-895-0582 / Outside US/Canada: (607) 772-6362
E-mail: getinfo@haworth.com
PLEASE PHOTOCOPY THIS FORM FOR YOUR PERSONAL USE.

BOF96

OVERSEAS DISTRIBUTORS OF HAWORTH PUBLICATIONS

AUSTRALIA
Edumedia
Level 1, 575 Pacific Highway
St. Leonards, Australia 2065
(mail only) PO Box 1201
Crows Nest, Australia 2065
Tel: (61) 2 9901–4217 / Fax: (61) 2 9906-8465

CANADA
Haworth/Canada
450 Tapscott Road, Unit 1
Scarborough, Ontario M1B 5W1
Canada
(Mail correspondence and orders only. No returns or telephone inquiries. Canadian currency accepted.)

DENMARK, FINLAND, ICELAND, NORWAY & SWEDEN
Knud Pilegaard
Knud Pilegaard Marketing
Mindevej 45
DK-2860 Soborg, Denmark
Tel: (45) 396 92100

ENGLAND & UNITED KINGDOM
Alan Goodworth
Roundhouse Publishing Group
62 Victoria Road
Oxford OX2 7QD, U.K.
Tel: 44–1865–521682 / Fax: 44–1865-559594
E-mail: 100637.3571@CompuServe.com

GERMANY, AUSTRIA & SWITZERLAND
Bernd Feldmann
Heinrich Roller Strasse 21
D–10405 Berlin, Germany
Tel: (49) 304–434–1621 / Fax: (49) 304–434–1623
E-mail: BFeldmann@t-online.de

JAPAN
Mrs. Masako Kitamura
MK International, Ltd.
1–50–7–203 Itabashi
Itabashi–ku
Tokyo 173, Japan

KOREA
Se–Yung Jun
Information & Culture Korea
Suite 1016, Life Combi Bldg.
61–4 Yoido–dong
Seoul, 150–010, Korea

MEXICO, CENTRAL AMERICA & THE CARIBBEAN
Mr. L.D. Clepper, Jr.
PMRA: Publishers Marketing & Research Association
P.O. Box 720489
Jackson Heights, NY 11372 USA
Tel/Fax: (718) 803–3465
E-mail: clepper@usa.pipeline.com

NEW ZEALAND
Brick Row Publishing Company, Ltd.
Attn: Ozwald Kraus
P.O. Box 100–057
Auckland 10, New Zealand
Tel/Fax: (64) 09–410–6993

PAKISTAN
Tahir M. Lodhi
Al-Rehman Bldg., 2nd Fl.
P.O. Box 2458
65–The Mall
Lahore 54000, Pakistan
Tel/Fax: (92) 42–724–5007

PEOPLE'S REPUBLIC OF CHINA & HONG KONG
Mr. Thomas V. Cassidy
Cassidy and Associates
470 West 24th Street
New York, NY 10011 USA
Tel: (212) 727–8943 / Fax: (212) 727–8539

PHILIPPINES, GUAM & PACIFIC TRUST TERRITORIES
I.J. Sagun Enterprises, Inc.
Tony P. Sagun
2 Topaz Rd. Greenheights Village
Ortigas Ave. Extension Tatay, Rizal
Republic of the Philippines
P.O. Box 4322 (Mailing Address)
CPO Manila 1099
Tel/Fax: (63) 2–658–8466

SOUTH AMERICA
Mr. Julio Emöd
PMRA: Publishers Marketing & Research Assoc.
Rua Joauim Tavora 629
São Paulo, SP 04015001 Brazil
Tel: (55) 11 571–1122 / Fax: (55) 11 575-6876

SOUTHEAST ASIA & THE SOUTH PACIFIC, SOUTH ASIA, AFRICA & THE MIDDLE EAST
The Haworth Press, Inc.
Margaret Tatich, Sales Manager
10 Alice Street
Binghamton, NY 13904–1580 USA
Tel: (607) 722–5857 ext. 321 / Fax: (607) 722–3487
E-mail: getinfo@haworth.com

RUSSIA & EASTERN EUROPE
International Publishing Associates
Michael Gladishev
International Publishing Associates
c/o Mazhdunarodnaya Kniga
Bolshaya Yakimanka 39
Moscow 117049 Russia
Fax: (095) 251–3338
E-mail: russbook@online. ru

LATVIA, LITHUANIA & ESTONIA
Andrea Hedgecock
c/o Iki Tareikalavimo
Kaunas 2042
Lithuania
Tel/Fax: (370) 777-0241 / E-mail: andrea@soften.ktu.lt

SINGAPORE, TAIWAN, INDONESIA, THAILAND & MALAYSIA
Steven Goh
APAC Publishers
35 Tannery Rd.
#10–06, Tannery Block
Singapore, 1334
Tel: (65) 747–8662 / Fax: (65) 747–8916
E-mail: sgohapac@signet.com.sg